Palliative care cor
head and neck cancer

SERIES EDITOR

Sara Booth
Macmillan Consultant in Palliative Medicine
Lead Clinician in Palliative Care
Cambridge University Hospitals NHS Foundation Trust

and

Honorary Senior Lecturer
Department of Palliative Care and Policy
King's College London

OTHER BOOKS IN THE SERIES

Palliative care consultations in haemato-oncology
Palliative care consultations in gynaeoncology
Palliative care consultations in primary and metastatic brain tumours
Palliative care consultations in advanced breast cancer

Palliative care consultations in head and neck cancer

Edited by

Sara Booth
Macmillan Consultant in Palliative Medicine
and Director of the Palliative Care Service,
Addenbrooke's Palliative Care Team,
Cambridge, UK

and

Andrew Davies
Consultant in Palliative Medicine,
Royal Marsden Hospital NHS Foundation Trust,
Sutton, UK

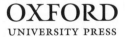

OXFORD
UNIVERSITY PRESS

OXFORD
UNIVERSITY PRESS

Great Clarendon Street, Oxford ox2 6DP

Oxford University Press is a department of the University of Oxford.
It furthers the University's objective of excellence in research, scholarship,
and education by publishing worldwide in

Oxford New York

Auckland Cape Town Dar es Salaam Hong Kong Karachi
Kuala Lumpur Madrid Melbourne Mexico City Nairobi
New Delhi Shanghai Taipei Toronto

With offices in

Argentina Austria Brazil Chile Czech Republic France Greece
Guatemala Hungary Italy Japan Poland Portugal Singapore
South Korea Switzerland Thailand Turkey Ukraine Vietnam

Oxford is a registered trade mark of Oxford University Press
in the UK and in certain other countries

Published in the United States
by Oxford University Press Inc., New York

British Library Cataloguing in Publication Data

Data available

Library of Congress Cataloging-in-Publication Data

Data available

Typeset by SPI Publisher Services, Pondicherry, India
Printed in Great Britain
on acid-free paper by
Biddles Ltd., King's Lynn, Norfolk

ISBN 10: 0–19–853074–9 (Paperback)
ISBN 13: 978–0–19–853074–9 (Paperback)

1 3 5 7 9 10 8 6 4 2

Series Foreword

Despite the significant advances in diagnosis and treatment that have been made in recent decades, cancer remains a major cause of death in all developed countries. It is therefore essential that all health professionals who provide direct care for cancer patients should be aware of what can be done to alleviate suffering.

Major progress has been made over the past thirty years or so in the relief of physical symptoms and in approaches to the delivery of psychological, social, and spiritual care for cancer patients and their families and carers. However, the problems of providing holistic care should not be underestimated. This is particularly the case in busy acute general hospitals and cancer centres. The physical environment may not be conducive to the care of a dying patient. Staff may have difficulty recognizing the point at which radical interventions are no longer in a patient's best interests, when the emphasis should change to care with palliative intent.

Progress in the treatment of cancer has also led to many patients who, although incurable, living for years with their illness. They may have repeated courses of treatment and some will have a significant burden of symptoms that must be optimally controlled.

One of the most important developments in recent years has been the recognition of the benefits of a multidisciplinary or multiprofessional approach to cancer care. Physicians, surgeons, radiologists, haematologists, pathologists, oncologists, palliative care specialists, nurse specialists, and a wide range of other health professionals all have major contributions to make. These specialists need to work together in teams.

One of the prerequisites for effective teamwork is that individual members should recognize the contribution that others can make. The *Palliative Care Consultations* series should help to make this a reality. The editors are to be congratulated in bringing together distinguished cancer and palliative care specialists from all parts of the world. Individual volumes focus predominantly on the problems faced by patients with a particular type of cancer (e.g. breast or lung) or groups of cancers (e.g. haematological malignancies or gynaecological cancers). The chapters of each volume set out what can be achieved using anticancer treatments and through the delivery of palliative care.

I warmly welcome the series and I believe the individual volumes will prove valuable to a wide range of clinicians involved in the delivery of high quality care.

Professor M. A. Richards
National Cancer Director, England

Contents

List of Contributors

Martin Birchall
Professor of Laryngology and
Consultant in Otorhinolaryngology
and Head and Neck Cancer,
University of Bristol, UK

Sara Booth
Macmillan Consultant in Palliative
Medicine and Director, Palliative
Care Services, Addenbrooke's NHS
Trust, Cambridge, UK

Frances M.B. Calman
Consultant Clinical Oncologist
Guy's and St Thomas' Cancer Centre,
London, UK

Andrew Davies
Consultant in Palliative Medicine
Royal Marsden Hospital NHS
Foundation Trust,
Sutton, UK

Maria Frampton
Consultant Psychiatrist,
St Luke's Hospital,
Kilkenny, Ireland

Nicholas Gibbins
Addenbrooke's Hospital,
Cambridge, UK

Neil A. Hagen
Professor, Department of Oncology,
Clinical Neurosciences and
Medicine, University of Calgary,
Canada

Piyush Jani
Addenbrooke's Hospital,
Cambridge, UK

Diane Laverty
Clinical Nurse Specialist in Palliative
Care, The Royal Marsden NHS
Foundation Trust, London and
Surrey, UK

Declan Lyons
Consultant Psychiatrist, St Patrick's
Hospital, Dublin, Ireland; Lecturer in
Psychiatry, Trinity College, Dublin,
Ireland

Jane Machin
formerly Specialist Speech and
Language Therapist, Royal Marsden
Hospital NHS Foundation Trust,
London and Surrey, UK

Clare Shaw
Consultant Dietician, The Royal
Marsden NHS Foundation Trust,
London and Surrey, UK

Fabian Sipaul
Specialist Registrar in
Otorhinolaryngology and Head and
Neck Surgery, Southmead Hospital,
Bristol, UK

Emma Thompson
Specialist Registrar in Palliative
Medicine, Royal Marsden Hospital
NHS Foundation Trust, Sutton, UK

Denise Traue
Macmillan Consultant in Palliative
Medicine, Addenbrooke's Hospital,
Cambridge University Hospitals
NHS Foundation Trust, UK

Marc Webster
Assistant Professor, Department of
Oncology, University of Calgary,
Canada

Chapter 1

Introduction

Denise Traue and Sara Booth

'Head and neck cancer' is an umbrella term which encompasses a diverse group of tumours that arise from the epithelial lining of the upper aerodigestive tract. It includes tumours of the oral cavity, salivary glands, paranasal sinuses, larynx, and pharynx. The histology of more than 90% of these tumours is of the squamous cell type.

The global incidence is around 500 000 new cases per year and it continues to rise.[1] Head and neck cancers are relatively uncommon in the Western world, constituting only 3–4% of new cancer diagnoses per year in the UK, although across the world they form the sixth most common tumour group. However, their relatively low incidence does not reflect the frequency with which patients are seen by palliative care services.

One of the most significant aetiological factors in the development of head and neck cancers is tobacco use, by either smoking or chewing. Alcohol ingestion is another major contributor and is synergistic when combined with tobacco use. The importance of these factors accounts for the disproportionately high percentage of male patients, and those from lower socioeconomic groups, which can make management more complicated. There are also important racial/ethnic factors to account for some of the variation in incidence. For example, carcinoma of the nasopharynx related to Epstein–Barr virus (EBV) has a significantly higher occurrence in oriental populations, and the use of betel nut in Asian populations results in an increased occurrence of oral tumours.

Patients experience a unique constellation of symptoms associated with the anatomical relationship of the tumours to critical structures, and the concurrent psychosocial issues experienced by this patient group. Thus, as well as experiencing symptoms common to all cancer types (such as pain), head and neck cancer can affect the most fundamental activities of daily living, including speech, swallowing, hearing, and breathing. These problems are discussed in more detail in the following chapters. Whilst survival and recurrence statistics have traditionally been viewed as the paramount determinants in cancer management, increasing awareness of the importance of the behavioural and functional impact of treatment on patients has led to a move towards optimization of quality as well as quantity of life.

Treatment aimed at cure is usually multimodal, and these strategies are discussed further in Chapters 2 and 3. Early stage head and neck cancer has a good cure rate with local treatment; in contrast, advanced disease has a poor response rate to standard treatment modalities including surgery, chemotherapy, and radiotherapy. All these therapies can be associated with substantial treatment-related morbidities. Complications of surgery include pain and discomfort, tightness, altered sensation, weakness, and sometimes significant disfigurement. Indeed, these procedures may have an adverse effect on daily life for about a third of patients—the proportion is higher in those groups with more advanced disease or also treated with radiotherapy and chemotherapy.[2,3] Radiotherapy, used either alone or in combination, also has significant related morbidities, including pain, mucositis, xerostomia, osteoradionecrosis, and subcutaneous fibrosis. The importance of multiprofessional working, coupled with excellent communication with patient and family in order to make the right treatment decisions for the patient's quality of life, cannot be overemphasized.

The complex physical symptoms experienced by head and neck cancer patients, in conjunction with the psychosocial issues experienced, mean that patients have a considerable need for holistic palliative care. This should be integrated into patient care from diagnosis, as input is required at all stages of the disease journey to assist in the management of tumour-related symptoms and the acute and long-term effects of disease-modifying therapies (even amongst patients who are receiving 'curative' treatment).

Speech

The ability to speak is one of the main prerequisites for communication and social interaction. Loss of this ability, therefore, has both important functional and psychological sequelae. The two speech components most affected by head and neck cancer and its treatment are intelligibility and voice quality. In general, the more extensive the disease and radical the treatment required, the greater the loss of function. Following laryngectomy, vocal and social rehabilitation are crucial. This involves development of oesophageal voice technique and good stoma care.

However, it is not solely the objective level of function that is important, but the individual patient's attitude towards and acceptance of that level of function. Personal reactions to functional status are not always strongly related to the specific level of impairment.[4] Whilst the majority of patients will eventually regain an adequate voice, some may need to use a vibrating 'artificial larynx', which may be socially unacceptable. In view of this, patient input concerning speech outcomes should be an important factor in choosing between available treatment options for head and neck cancer.

Swallowing and nutrition

Swallowing dysfunction is common with head and neck cancers, related to either the tumour itself or its management. Swallowing impairment impacts not only on nutritional status, but also psychologically as a result of the loss of the social aspect of eating. More advanced tumours and oropharyngeal lesions have the highest incidence of pre-treatment dysphagia.[5] Although swallowing difficulties may resolve after completion of the acute phase of treatment, for some patients this is a longer term problem.[6,7] The extent of surgical resection, particularly the amount of tongue removed, is the primary correlate of post-surgical swallowing dysfunction in oral and oropharyngeal tumours, with more extensive surgery resulting in a higher level of dysfunction. Mucositis and xerostomia can also reduce the ability to swallow,[8] and early recognition and good palliation of these problems can have both functional and quality of life benefits.

Nutritional deficits have a high incidence in both newly diagnosed patients and those with progressive disease. Early consideration must be given to how nutritional requirements will be met. Where severe swallowing dysfunction already exists, or is likely to develop during treatment, options for artificial feeding should be considered such as PEG (percutaneous endoscopic gastrostomy) feeding tube insertion.[9] Ensuring good nutritional support can decrease hospital stay and recovery time after treatment. Multidisciplinary input from dieticians and speech and language therapists is crucial from the time of diagnosis onwards to optimize quality of life and enable patients to tolerate treatment.

Xerostomia and mucositis

Xerostomia, or dry mouth, can occur from a variety of causes. It is a common problem following radiotherapy to the oral cavity, affecting the majority of patients treated to some extent.[10] With the combined use of chemo-radiation, the severity of the problem is increased.[11] Drugs commonly used in symptom control, such as opioid analgesics and tricyclic antidepressants, can also exacerbate the problem.

Dry mouth may result in a number of other problems, including oral discomfort, altered taste sensation, impaired swallowing, speech problems, dental caries, and other oral infections. Because of these factors, xerostomia can have a major impact on quality of life. Nutritional status and even continuation with disease-modifying therapy can be affected.[12] Consideration of treatment modalities to spare salivary gland function, as well as early recognition and treatment of xerostomia when it occurs, is crucial to minimize morbidity and maintain quality of life.

Oral and pharyngeal mucositis can occur as an acute response to both radiotherapy and chemotherapy. It is a distressing and debilitating problem, resulting in pain that may be difficult to control, and dysfunction in swallowing and speech. Stringent use of mouth care regimens during and after treatment may reduce symptoms. However, in severe cases, patients may require hospitalization for administration of parenteral hydration and analgesia.

Pain

One of the most important symptomatic problems in head and neck cancer is pain. The pain is often of a mixed aetiology, and may be caused by the tumour itself or the treatments used in disease management. It is also a multidimensional phenomenon, with biological and psychological factors interacting.

Tumour-related pain is a common feature at presentation, affecting 50–80% of patients.[13] Tumour pain is often a combination of soft tissue, bone, and neuropathic pain.[14] Ulceration of mucosa may result in inflammation, oedema, and infection all causing pain. Bony involvement and direct invasion or compression of neural structures also contributes. The temporal nature of the pain is variable; as well as continuous background pain, there is often incident pain, related to oral intake or speech. Pain becomes an increasing problem in more advanced disease, where prevalence increases to 80–100%.[14]

Whilst disease-modifying treatment may be beneficial in reducing tumour-related pain, it may also result in the development of new pain problems. Both acute and chronic pains are a common problem after surgery for head and neck cancer, due to damaged nerves, structural misalignment, and dysfunction.[15,16] There is also a variation in pain over time, with head and neck pain decreasing after surgery, but shoulder pain becoming more prevalent.[14] Radiotherapy side effects such as mucositis, xerostomia, osteoradionecrosis, and subcutaneous fibrosis also cause pain and discomfort.

Irrespective of the cause of pain, it has a negative impact on function and quality of life. Specialist drug management as well as physical therapy to maintain function are key. Achieving good pain management is challenging in this population not only because of the complex pathophysiology of the pain, but also because of the associated psychosocial factors. These issues are often inextricably linked, and the concept of total pain must be addressed to enable adequate symptom control. Specialist input is essential to optimize pain management and quality of life.

Airway obstruction and haemorrhage

Due to their location, head and neck cancers may result in airway compromise. Impingement on respiratory structures can result in dyspnoea and fatigue. More advanced tumours can result in critical obstruction necessitating tracheostomy insertion. Ideally, patients at risk of developing obstruction should be identified and elective tracheostomy insertion performed, since a planned procedure has lower associated morbidity than one performed as an emergency. Multiprofessional input with advice on tracheostomy care and speech therapy are integral parts of ongoing care.

Vascular structures are at risk not just from local tumour invasion, but also as a result of surgery or radiotherapy. Carotid artery rupture or 'blow out' is an uncommon but catastrophic occurrence. In patients undergoing active management, urgent treatment is needed with interventional radiology or surgery. In the palliative setting, management with sedation and analgesia, if required, may be the preferred option.

It is important to identify patients at risk of airway obstruction or haemorrhage to enable sensitive discussion in advance of any acute event. Patients would then be able to consider what their treatment wishes would be in light of disease stage and prognosis, i.e. either active management (such as tracheostomy insertion) or palliation. If these discussions are left until a crisis occurs, the patient may not be able to participate in decision-making processes, and unwanted interventions may be performed.

Psychosocial factors

Although most patients will successfully adapt to their diagnosis and treatment in the longer term, many will experience mood disturbances, including depression and anxiety, at some stage of their illness.[17] A holistic approach to patient care, including a heightened awareness of the risk of psychological problems and optimization of symptom control, may enable 'at risk' patients to be identified earlier so that intervention can be initiated to ameliorate long-term problems.

Depression is a common reaction to cancer, but head and neck patients are particularly vulnerable due to the combination of physical, functional, and psychological sequelae of the disease and its management.[5] Around 30% of patients with head and neck cancer experience depression, and this can persist for months to several years after treatment.[19,20] Untreated depression has a significant impact on multiple aspects of a patient's life, resulting in prolonged hospital admissions, higher incidence of treatment-related complications, impaired ability to care for oneself, and a general decrease in quality of life.[21]

Disfigurement is recognized as one of the most significant factors influencing the psychological response of patients. This is because of the importance of facial appearance to self-image, esteem, communication, and interpersonal relationships.[22] Undergoing treatment, including surgery and radiotherapy, increases low mood, and the presence of higher levels of dysfunction and physical symptoms such as pain are also important predictors for psychological distress. There is also a gender variation in psychological distress, with greater anxiety and depression in women, partly related to the higher importance placed on physical appearance.[22] Patients from low socio-economic classes also have a higher risk of depression.[23]

The presence of effective coping mechanisms and good social support protect against psychological problems.[18,19] However, the chaotic lifestyle of some head and neck patients, associated with alcohol use, may mean that these protective frameworks are often absent. Moreover, the tendency of patients to blame themselves for their illness, with patients attributing the cause of their condition to their own past actions of alcohol and tobacco use, can result in a substantially increased risk of depression.[23] Head and neck cancer may also reduce patients' financial resources, with over half of patients unable to return to work after treatment.[13]

Conclusion

Head and neck cancer patients experience a complex constellation of physical symptoms and psychosocial problems. The psychosocial variables are as important as the physiological ones in determining quality of life, making a holistic approach an essential part of care throughout the disease course, from diagnosis to cure or the end of life. Provision of palliative care should, therefore, be viewed as an integral component of the management of patients with head and neck cancers. This book has been based on these principles, and each of the components of excellent multidisciplinary care is addressed in detail by leaders in their respective field.

References

1 Souhami, R., and Tobias, J. (eds) (2005). *Cancer and its management*, 5th edn. Oxford, Blackwell Publishing.

2 Shah, S., Gady, H., and Rosenfeld, R. (2001). Short-term and long-term quality of life after neck dissection. *Head Neck*, **23**, 954–961.

3 Jalukar, V., Funk, G., Christiansen, A., Hynds Karnell, L., and Moran, P. (1998). Health states following head and neck cancer treatment: patient, health-care professional and public perspectives. *Head Neck*, 20, 600–608.

4 Hynds Karnell, L., Funk, G., Tomblin, B., and Hoffman, H. (1999). Quality of life measurements of speech in the head and neck cancer population. *Head Neck*, 21, 229–238.

5 Pauloski, B., Rademaker, A., Logemann, J., *et al.* (2000). Pre-treatment swallowing function in patients with head and neck cancer. *Head Neck* 22, 474–482.

6 Hughes, P., Scott, P., Kew, J., *et al.* (2000). Dysphagia in treated nasopharyngeal cancer. *Head Neck*, 22, 393–397.

7 Kotz, T., Costello, R., Li, Y., and Posner, M. (2004). Swallowing dysfunction after chemoradiation for advanced squamous cell carcinoma of the head and neck. *Head Neck*, 26, 365–372.

8 Pauloski, B., Rademaker, A., Logemann, J., *et al.* (2004). Surgical variables affecting swallowing in patients treated for oral/oropharyngeal cancer *Head Neck*, 26, 625–636.

9 Schweinfurth, J., Boger, G., and Feustel, P. (2001). Preoperative risk assessment for gastrostomy tube placement in head and neck cancer patients. *Head Neck*, 23, 376–382.

10 Wijers, O., Levendag, P., Braaksma, M., *et al.* (2002). Patients with head and neck cancer cured by radiation therapy: a survey of the dry mouth syndrome in long-term survivors. *Head Neck*, 24, 737–747.

11 Logemann, J., Smith, C., Pauloski, B., *et al.* (2001). Effects of xerostomia on perception and performance of swallow function. *Head Neck*, 23, 317–321.

12 Chambers, M., Garden, A., Kies, M., and Martin, J. (2004). Radiation-induced xerostomia in patients with head and neck cancer: pathogenesis, impact on quality of life, and management. *Head Neck*, 26, 796–807.

13 Doyle, D., Hanks, G., Cherny, N., and Calman, K. (eds) (2005). *Oxford textbook of palliative medicine*, 3rd edn. Oxford, Oxford University Press.

14 Chaplin, J., and Morton, R. (1999). A prospective, longitudinal study of pain in head and neck cancer patients. *Head Neck*, 21, 531–537.

15 Dijkstra, P., Wilgen, P., Buijs, R., *et al.* (2001). Incidence of shoulder pain after neck dissection: a clinical explorative study for risk factors. *Head Neck*, 23, 947–953.

16 Wilgen, C., Dijkstra, P., ven der Lann, B., *et al.* (2004). Morbidity of the neck after head and neck cancer therapy. *Head Neck*, 26, 785–791.

17 Holloway, R., Hellewell, J., Marbella, A., Layde, P., Myers, K., and Campbell, B. (2005). Psychosocial effects in long-term head and neck cancer survivors. *Head Neck*, 27, 281–288.

18 De Leeuw, J., De Graeff, A., Ros, W., Blijham, G., Hordijk, G., and Winnubst, J. (2000). Prediction of depressive symptomatology after treatment for head and neck cancer: the influence of pre-treatment physical and depressive symptoms, coping and social support, *Head Neck*, 22, 799–807.

19 De Leeuw, J., De Graeff, A., Ros, W., Blijham, G., Hordijk, G., and Winnubst, J. (2001). Prediction of depression 6 months to 3 years after treatment of head and neck cancer. *Head Neck*, 23, 892–898.

20 Rapoport, Y., Kreitler, S., Chaitchik, S., Algor, R., and Weissler, K. (1993). Psychosocial problems in head and neck cancer patients and their change with time since diagnosis. *Ann Oncol*, 4, 69–73.

21 McDaniel, J.S., Dominique, L., Musselman, L., *et al.* (1995). Depression in patients with cancer. Diagnosis, biology and treatment. *Arch Gen Psychiatry*, **52**, 89–99.

22 Katz, M., Irish, J., Devins, G., Rodin, G., and Gullane, P. (2003). Psychosocial adjustment in head and neck cancer: the impact of disfigurement, gender and social support. *Head Neck*, **25**, 103–112.

23 Sehlen, S., Lenk, M., Herschbach, P., *et al.* (2003). Depressive symptoms during and after radiotherapy for head and neck cancer. *Head Neck*, **25**, 1004–1018.

Chapter 2

Surgery with palliative intent in advanced or recurrent head and neck cancer

Fabian Sipaul and Martin Birchall

Summary

Surgery is an important, but often underused part of the head and neck palliative care armamentarium. This is not surprising, as the morbidity of surgery can be considerable. Nonetheless, there are a number of areas of the palliative care of the patient with head and neck cancer to which surgery may contribute. Surgical relief of symptoms ranges from tracheostomy to allow adequate breathing, to simple reduction in tumour bulk, to complex procedures with reconstruction. Site-specific management issues, including prevention of complications during surgery with curative intent, are also important to optimize quality of life for the patient. The correct application of these techniques is often hampered by a bilateral failure of understanding between surgical and palliative care teams about how much the other has to offer. As head and neck cancer patients are, arguably, more in need of palliative input than those with a tumour at any other site, the case for inclusion of palliative care team members in the multidisciplinary team and treatment planning in every centre is, in our opinion, overwhelming. More funding is needed to make this happen, and clinical trials are needed to establish the true worth of surgical techniques in advanced disease.

Introduction

Broadly speaking, the term advanced cancer means either that the cancer has a high volume, that it has involved bone or vital surrounding structures, or that it has spread beyond the primary site. According to the latest audit of head and neck cancer in the UK,[1] one-third of newly presenting head and neck cancers are tumour stage T3 or T4,[2] one-third have nodal metastases and 3% have distant metastases at presentation. However, this only tells part of the story, as 40% of the workload of head and neck cancer units involves the management of recurrent disease, most of which are at an advanced stage. Depending on the site and histological features, long-term (>5 years) patient survival is possible for about 30% of these patients. However, for the majority, failure to clear primary disease or recurrent disease will mean that patients have symptoms usually localized to the head and neck region until eventually death supervenes. The results of extensive surgery or combined treatment, particularly chemo-radiation, can still lead to intractable symptoms for survivors. These symptoms can severely affect quality of life, even without the clinical presence of the tumour.

Surgery, radiotherapy, and synchronous chemotherapy and radiotherapy are the mainstays of curative treatment of head and neck cancer. Each has an important part to play in control of symptoms and maintenance of the patient's quality of life for as long as possible. Whilst the roles of radiotherapy and chemotherapy have been reasonably well delineated, as described elsewhere in this book, the place of surgery in this setting is rarely considered. There are hardly any national guidelines that exist for its correct application. Yet, even complex surgery with reconstruction may be the best form of palliation in advanced cases. Indeed, it could be argued that the prognosis for the worst forms of disease is so poor that surgeons are deluding themselves if they believe that some operations are anything other than palliative. The palliative care services in many countries including the UK are still based on outdated models of care and culture. The provision and funding of palliative care services in the UK is at best patchy. As a result, there is often inadequate communication between palliative care teams and the surgeons who tend to dominate treatment planning discussions in most centres. A balanced discussion of the role of surgery in so-called 'incurable' disease, or in those with intractable symptoms, is long overdue.

Aims of the chapter

1 To provide an overview of surgery with palliative intent in clinical practice, based on literature review (Medline and Cochrane databases).

2 To review current debate/controversies regarding the role of surgery as palliation in head and neck cancer.

3 To review common and specific problems in surgery for palliation in head and neck cancer and highlight difficult symptoms/problems and possible ways of managing them.

Role of surgery in the control of symptoms

Managing pain

Whilst much can be accomplished to reduce pain pharmacologically or with skilled application of radiotherapy to advanced head and neck cancers, the management of pain might be regarded as one of the primary goals of major surgical removal of bulky disease. Since resection of the most advanced tumours is often associated with positive margins and poor prognosis, the biggest operations could technically be regarded as palliative in most cases, even if the team involved find it difficult to admit. Hence, philosophically, the control of pain and other symptoms could easily be placed ahead of 'cure' in the surgical goals of treating advanced head and neck cancer.

Head and neck surgery has been regarded by some as principally surgery of the *nerves* of the head and neck. These are responsible for both pain and function. Thus, avoidance of nerve damage where possible is a primary goal. The surgeon may be torn between respecting an obviously involved vagus nerve for example: on the one hand, this might give him better 'clearance' of tumour and a remote possibility of elusive 'cure'; on the other hand, the chances of long-term survival are so poor that it could be argued that preservation of speech and swallowing for the remaining lifespan is more important. How a clinician approaches dilemmas like this depends on a combination of training[3] and selection based on knowledge of that patient's individual characteristics and personality.

'Preventative' surgery can also help to minimize pain later on. Avoidance of damage to sensory nerves during resection can prevent development of neuromas and some neuropathic pain. Shoulder pain is the symptom that most patients complain about following neck dissection and is related to a combination of accessory nerve damage/resection and scarring. Preservation of the accessory nerve and avoidance of dissecting any more levels of the neck than is absolutely necessary are therefore crucial principles, as is post-operative physiotherapy.[4]

Careful design of incisions will reduce contractures. Nonetheless, even when incisions and dissection have been performed carefully, the application of adjuvant radiotherapy and especially chemo-radiation can still cause severe scarring, tightness, and pain. Where shoulder pain is related to tight scarring, division of contractures can be performed. The introduction of Z-plasties into linear scars can remove tension and improve appearance. Occasionally, severe contractures will benefit from division and subsequent application of a skin graft.

Improving communication

Contact between the soft palate and posterior pharyngeal wall is important in articulation of 'plosive' consonants such as b, d, g, k, p, t, ch, and sh. In patient with unilateral palatal paralysis, the patient's speech can be hypernasal in quality and can be unintelligible if severe.[5] Vocal volume is softer because as much as 10 dB of sound is lost through the nose.[6] When cancer dictates surgical resection of the soft palate, the resulting deficit creates a velopharyngeal gap and thus insufficiency. Similarly, tumour involvement or its removal may require disruption of the glossopharyngeal and vagus nerves. The resulting unilateral paralysis causes a velopharyngeal gap. When the gap is minimal, behavioural therapy may facilitate over-articulation of speech sounds, which may be sufficient to reduce nasality and improve intelligibility.[7] However, surgery may be warranted for larger defects. Posterior pharyngeal wall implants may be used, such as silicone or collagen. This allows the posterior pharyngeal wall to be in contact with the soft palate during its elevation. Migration of these substances, although less of a problem than it was formerly with Teflon, remains a concern[8,9]

The most popular surgery is the creation of a pharyngeal flap by suturing a superiorly based flap from the posterior pharyngeal wall to the soft palate to bridge the space. In the case of palatal paralysis following involvement or sacrifice of the vagus nerve for skull base tumours, a palatal adhesion eliminates hypernasality and nasal regurgitation. The paralysed side of the soft palate is sutured to the posterior pharyngeal wall to close the gap between the oral and nasal cavities.[10]

Despite the widespread use of advanced reconstructive techniques, especially free tissue transfer, surgery and/or chemo-radiation may lead to tethering of the tongue or other oral structures. This may be corrected by division and insertion of fresh tissue, either free or revascularized.[11,12]

In the palliative setting, bilateral cord paralysis either due to the effect of malignancy or as a complication of surgery usually results in difficulty in breathing which is manifested by noisy inspiratory/expiratory noise, i.e. stridor. This is probably best managed by tracheostomy and is covered in Chapter 4. Voice is not the major issue here, particularly since the cords are generally both lying in a paramedian position enabling reasonable sound generation. Rarely, it is necessary to perform total laryngectomy to remove the disability of a larynx, which no longer functions.

In patients with unilateral impairment of vocal fold function, a breathy and diplophonic voice impairs communication. In addition, the enlarged posterior glottic gap and differing heights of the vocal cords combine with changes in sensation to produce both aspiration and weakness of coughing. This disability may result from paralysis of recurrent laryngeal nerve or involvement of the vagus nerve by tumour or operation, or it may result from partial laryngeal surgery such as laser resection. For these patients, medialization laryngoplasty can be very beneficial. This procedure repositions the immobile vocal fold into a more favourable midline position and allows contact with the other mobile vocal fold. Most commonly, an injectable substance such as collagen or synthetics (e.g. Bioplastique) is placed using either local (percutaneous or flexible endoscopic routes) or general anaesthetic. Sufficient material is injected lateral to the cord to push the free vibrating edges close together, with great improvement in voice and cough strength.

A more precise result may be obtained using laryngeal framework surgery under sedation. Here, an incision is made over the lateral aspect of the thyroid cartilage and various materials (presently Gore-tex and silastic are most popular) are placed to splint the vocal cord closer to the midline. The addition of cricothyroid approximation[13] and arytenoid medialization techniques[14] gives a superior vocal result to simple injection, as these procedures are able to correct the coronal height of the cord as well as its sagittal alignment (Fig. 2.1). Not surprisingly, they are more time-consuming and require greater

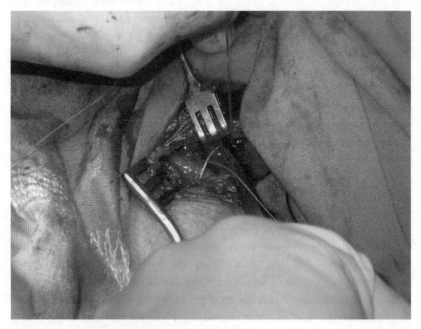

Fig. 2.1 Vocal cord medialization: exposure of the arytenoid cartilage for closure of the posterior commissure.

expertise. Studies have documented that voice quality is better or normal following phonosurgery.[15]

It should be said that any attempt to improve phonation by surgery is incomplete without the involvement of specialist speech and swallowing therapists to maximize the result. Indeed, surgery should only be used in the palliative setting where it is felt that the speech and swallowing team has already achieved as much as possible and yet significant residual disability remains.

Managing problems with deglutition and swallowing

Difficulties with deglutition and swallowing are common in advanced head and neck cancer, especially in the palliative setting. Dysphagia or odynophagia (painful swallowing) may either be due to advanced or recurrent cancer or as a result of cancer treatment (particularly chemo-radiotherapy). This leads to malnutrition and weight loss. It should be assessed in a multidisciplinary manner by speech and swallowing therapists, dietitians, surgeons, and the palliative care team. Videofluoroscopy, FEES (functional endoscopic evaluation of swallowing), and bed-side testing are all important in gauging severity and response to treatment. This is covered in greater details in Chapter 6.

Where simple measures such as alternative swallowing strategies and altered food consistencies are inadequate, the most common approach to this problem is the provision of alternative routes of nutrition. Nasogastric tubes should only be used if the period of dysphagia is expected to be brief (≤ 2 weeks). All other cases should be considered for alternative tube insertion: percutaneous endoscopic gastrostomy (PEG), radiologically inserted gastrostomy (RIG), or jejunostomy may all be used. They are not without complications, including death from peritonitis. However, in experienced hands, the morbidity is low.[16,17] The post-operative care of such tubes needs specialist assistance. Community nurses and dietitians should be involved to help the patient and carers manage feeding at home as far as possible.

Where swallowing is impaired due to high strictures, dilatation may be performed under local (using flexible endoscopes) or general anaesthetic. If the problem is thought to be due to spasm or tightness of muscles as assessed clinically and/or by videofluoroscopy and especially where this involves the crico-pharyngeus, this may be addressed either by injection of botulinum toxin ('medical myotomy') locally or, if this fails, by surgical myotomy.

Extensive unresectable tumour recurrences within the pharynx may cause dysphagia, as well as airway problems and dysphonia. Sometimes, it is possible to perform trans-oral laser or diathermy resection of tumour mass to improve swallowing and other symptoms (Fig. 2.2a–c). This needs to be managed with

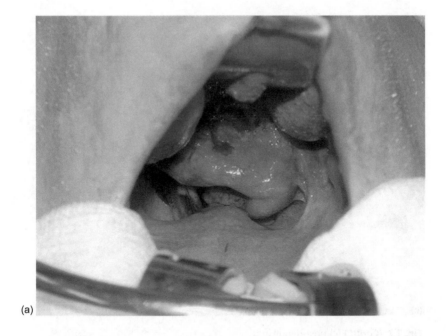

(a)

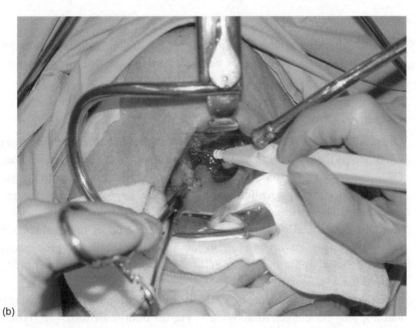

(b)

Fig. 2.2 Debulking of an oropharyngeal tumour with pen diathermy. (a) Pre-debulking; (b) during debulking; (c) post-debulking.

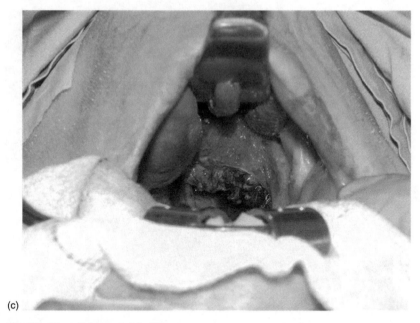
(c)

Fig. 2.2 (*Contd.*) (c) post-debulking.

care and with appropriate instrumentation for dealing with haemorrhage, which can be severe. Nonetheless, selected cases can get considerable symptomatic relief in this way.[18]

Osteoradionecrosis

Osteoradionecrosis (ORN) is one of the most dreaded complications from radiotherapy to the head and neck region. Fortunately it is a rare complication. ORN can result in exposure of bone, fistula formation, or pathological fracture. Therefore, prevention is of paramount importance. The current practice of dental clearance or selected extraction of diseased teeth by a specialist dentist and primary closure of the mucosa under minimal tension before the cancer surgery is done to minimize this. Antibiotic prophylaxis should be used, and a minimum of 14 days should be allowed for healing prior to use of radiation.[19]

The first line of treatment for established ORN is improving oral hygiene and stopping alcohol and tobacco use.[20] The use of hyperbaric oxygen (HBO) treatment for ORN has increased recently. There is good retrospective evidence of its effectiveness. However, prospective trials have so far been very small,[21] and a substantive randomized trial is urgently needed. Where these measures are unsuccessful or in severe primary cases, which can be highly painful, surgery to remove the affected bone, with or without adjuvant HBO, may be used. Surgery may involve resection using tetracycline fluorescence under ultraviolet light or until the presence of bleeding bone is seen to determine a healthy margin.[22] Stabilization of the mandible with either an extraskeletal pin or maxillofacial fixation is usually necessary before HBO therapy and reconstruction if required.

The airway

Maintenance of an airway is of primary importance in the head and neck cancer patient, and may be compromised either by disease or by its treatment (e.g. stenotic larynges after chemo-radiation, or alternative airways after laryngectomy). This subject is covered in detail in Chapter 4. Needless to say, surgery has a major role to play in establishing and maintaining a viable airway.

In brief, tracheostomies may be used to by-pass obstructions, although they often come at the considerable cost of worsened swallowing, speech, and aspiration. Choice of tube is important and depends on the balance required between these various functions. Specialist head and neck nurse involvement is crucial to a long-lasting good airway in all cases. Tumours obstructing the airway may be cleared by open surgery or by endoscopic excision, particularly with laser (Fig. 2.3a and b). Subglottic stenoses may also be dilated.

Altered body image

Many patients with advanced head and neck disease will require a form of feeding tube and/or a tracheostomy, which may be temporary or permanent. Some will have significant disfigurement of the face and neck. Studies suggest that the psychological impact of disease and treatment is generally underestimated,[23] and it is not uncommon for patients to venture outside the home only when they have to go to hospital. Altered body image affects many activities including socialization and sexuality. Laryngectomees not only have obvious changes in communication, but also have an altered ability to express emotions (laughing/crying) and even to kiss (as no air passes between the lips). These issues are dealt with primarily in Chapter 10, but surgeons can help by first acknowledging that these are serious issues, and by secondly applying methods that will minimize disfigurement and disability wherever possible.

Disfigurement may be helped by minor surgical procedures, such as blepharoplasty or simple face-lifts to obviate the effects of facial nerve weakness for example. Z-plasties and other facial plastic surgical techniques can

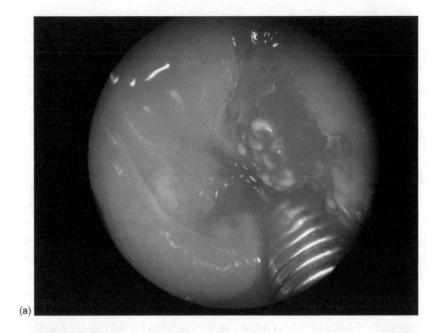

(a)

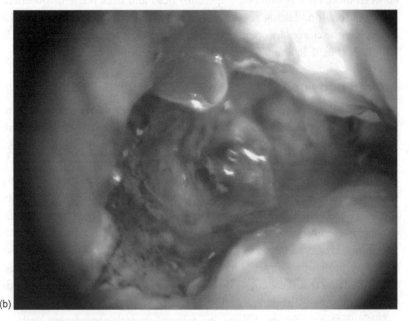

(b)

Fig. 2.3 Debulking of an airway-obstructing carcinoma with laser. (a) Pre-debulking; (b) post-debulking.

improve scar appearance. Although heroic changes to facial appearance are possible with surgery, these should only ever be considered when all prosthetic options have been tried. The quality of prosthetics, including the use of surgically inserted titanium implants, is now so good that major surgery should rarely be necessary especially in the palliative setting.[24]

Quality of life

There are a variety of validated tools now available for measuring quality of life in the surgical head and neck patient. Disease-specific measures are Functional Assessment of Cancer Therapy: Head & Neck Scale (FACT-H&N), University of Washington Quality of Life Scale (UW Qol), and European Organization for Research and Treatment of Cancer (EORTC-QLQ). FACT-H&N and EORTC QLQ have head and neck subscales, which address disease-specific symptoms.

There are no studies that we could find specifically addressing quality of life with respect to surgery for palliation. However, Goodwin[25] applied the Functioning Living Index For Cancer (FLIC) to 109 patients undergoing surgery for recurrent disease. He found that the efficacy of surgery in these cases was surprisingly good, with over 50% of patients reaching or exceeding their pre-operative FLIC scores. There was no effect of the interval between primary and recurrence on either FLIC changes or survival.

However, Goodwin's results were strongly stage dependent, with the most advanced recurrences resulting in a substantial loss of quality of life post-operatively compared with their pre-operative status, despite the removal of bulky and often painful tumours. As median survival was only 18 months for the whole group, any surgery for advanced recurrences must be considered largely palliative. In support of this, Goodwin also presented a meta-analysis of previous studies in the field with corroborative findings. The significant potential adverse effect on quality of life must enter into all discussions between multidisciplinary team members, patients, and carers.

The neck

Advanced neck disease

Advanced neck disease generally implies an International Union Against Cancer (UICC) staging of N2 or N3 (multiple, bilateral, contralateral, or massive lymph nodes).[2] The single best pathological predictor of poor outcome is extracapsular spread of tumour, and in the neck this can involve nerves, deep muscles, and great vessels. Current average 2-year survival rate associated with N3 (massive, >6 cm largest diameter) disease is only 15–20%, with a high rate of distant (mainly lung and liver) metastases. Management options for these patients are controversial. The goal of treatment in most of these cases is palliative, but cure can be possible.

Treatment of the primary tumour site usually dictates the plan for the neck. Clinical examination will reveal whether there is complete fixation, with involvement of deep neck musculature or great vessels. Imaging can evaluate the relationship of the tumour to the carotid artery and deep muscle, and help to evaluate the involvement of non-palpable nodes. The demonstration of normal tissue planes, particularly between posterior pharynx and pre-vertebral fascia/vertebral bodies, is crucial as involvement of either renders surgery with curative intent an impossibility.[26]

In Goodwin's study, overall quality of life and performance status was lower for patients with recurrent neck disease than for any other given primary site. Only 27% of patients with recurrent neck disease achieved or exceeded baseline FLIC following surgery, and even fewer regained baseline diet and public eating functions. This confirms the importance of fully evaluating and weighing neck disease before embarking on 'curative' surgery for advanced recurrent disease.

The great vessels

The jugular vein is often involved in neck node disease, which by definition must be extracapsular and therefore of poor prognosis in nature. Nonetheless, it is possible to remove one jugular vein with minimal morbidity. Synchronous removal of both veins may increase intracranial pressure significantly for a period and always results in disfiguring facial oedema, made more obvious by the removal of neck tissues. Thus, staged neck dissections are preferable in such cases.

Unlike the jugular vein, involvement of the carotid artery must be regarded as a sign of incurable disease. In cases where there is suspicion of carotid artery involvement by tumour, this can be confirmed by imaging, including dynamic techniques if available. Confirmation of carotid involvement makes curative resection of disease impossible.

Perhaps surprisingly, the issue of sacrifice of the internal or common carotid artery remains controversial. For example, Freeman[27] argued that the line separating attempted cure and palliative treatment is not as clear-cut as most other observers feel. Involvement of carotid arteries invariably implies involvement of other structures such as the sternocleidomastoid muscle, phrenic nerve, vagus nerve, internal jugular vein, base of skull, and scalene muscles. Resectability is a purely subjective opinion and in no cases implies cure. It is a radical approach to maintain local control, technically very demanding, and requires assistance from vascular and, occasionally, neurosurgical colleagues. Patients so treated rarely leave hospital.

Carotid resection may in exceptional circumstances be justified in order to reduce the risk of imminent and distressing 'blow out'. In these cases, pre-operative evaluation is vital to minimize mortality and neurological complications. Although balloon occlusion with electroencephalographic monitoring has been regarded as the gold standard, this is not without complications itself. Thus reliance has shifted to non-invasive measures such as functional magnetic resonance imaging (fMRI). Complications are less when vascular replacement by Dacron graft is performed. However, since this may result in the graft becoming exposed to more tumour, infection, and even the outside world, even fewer patients are suitable. When resection of the primary cancer requires pharyngotomy, vascular reconstruction is not recommended because contamination of the operative field and the possibility of a post-operative pharyngeal fistula produce a markedly increased risk of infection and graft disruption. As long-term control of disease in patients following carotid artery resection is extremely poor, placement of brachytherapy catheters into the surgical field may be considered. Such catheters may increase the risk of infection and anastomotic disruption if vascular grafting was performed. The severity of the resulting complications may shorten the life expectancy and reduce the quality of life for some patients. Thus the anticipated outcome must be carefully evaluated in and with each patient before proceeding with this form of surgery.[28]

More commonly, when the possibility of a major neck bleed is considered high, more conservative measures are taken. If there is a good possibility of getting the patient home, then a 'safe' flap, especially a pectoralis major musculocutaneous pedicled flap, to cover the at risk area may be considered. Where the neck is full of tumour, however, this is not feasible and prognosis is, in any case, measured in weeks at best. A decision is then made as to whether active treatment is required in the event of a bleed from the carotid (Fig. 2.4). This must be made in consultation with the patient and carers. If a patient at risk of a bleed is at home, then appropriate counselling of carers is necessary. Management of a bleed in a patient who is not for active treatment includes midazolam and analgesia as necessary. Green towels and sheets have been recommended to cover the area as these hide blood well and reduce the psychological impact slightly. Nonetheless, a carotid blow out is a shocking event, and counselling of relatives and even staff may be necessary afterwards.

Fungation

Fungation of cancer results in discharge, offensive smell, bleeding, pain, and cosmetic disfigurement. Surgery can be performed to treat or prevent fungation of cancer, even in a previously irradiated neck. Occasionally, palliative

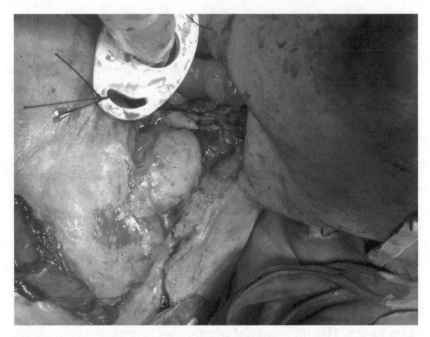

Fig. 2.4 Carotid artery blow out: managed with tying of the great vessels.

surgery is preferable to weeks of palliative radiotherapy. A patient can be out of the hospital in a matter of days. This is kept as simple as possible, with no concerns about margins. A simple shaving and skin grafting procedure may sometimes alleviate pain and the equally distressing discharge and smell (see also Chapter 8).

Site-specific issues in palliative surgery

Cancer of the larynx

In the UK, the policy in many centres is to irradiate virtually all tumours and to carry out a total laryngectomy for recurrent disease. This is acceptable treatment for small glottic tumours as the cure rate is high (80–90%). Open partial laryngeal surgery is not regarded as good treatment in a previously irradiated neck, though there have been series reporting reasonable control rates with salvage endoscopic laser surgery.[29] However, at the time of writing, there are no controlled prospective trials comparing radiotherapy with surgery for any site,[30] and the practice in other countries is very different. The main problem with salvage surgery is delayed or failed wound healing, although there is a slight trend towards a decrease in complications the longer the resection is performed from the time of completion of chemo-radiotherapy. Surgery that necessitates entry into the pharynx via the neck has higher complication rates, particularly from a pharyngo-cutaneous fistula. There is a suggestion that a more liberal use of vascularized flaps for reconstruction as opposed to primary closure may reduce this complication.[31]

As for recurrence after laryngectomy, radiotherapy and chemotherapy, alone or in combination, are the main treatment modalities. Tracheostomy may be required in patients with difficult airway where time may be gained to facilitate discussion with the relatives, to confirm the diagnosis, to allow the patient to come to terms with the situation, and also to secure the airway during further irradiation.[30]

A stoma in the neck is fashioned following total laryngectomy. The upper part of the trachea is connected to a hole in the neck to allow 'normal' breathing. Stomal recurrence presents a particular problem. Again, this is a particularly poor sign, and the presence of stomal disease during the terminal stages of laryngeal cancer is not uncommon (Fig. 2.5). Surgery is only really appropriate for the earliest type of stomal recurrence, for which a 45% 5-year survival has been reported.[32] The operation comprises excision of the lesion with an ellipse of skin around the stoma and reconstruction with regional skin

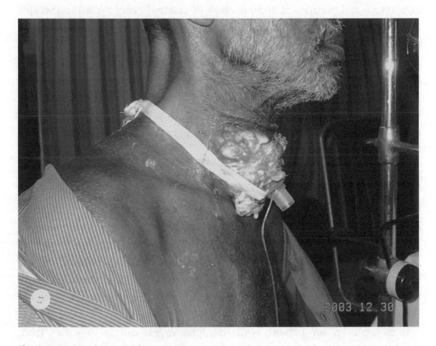

Fig. 2.5 Aggressive stomal recurrence.

flaps. However, in more extensive but resectable cases, regional myocutaneous flaps or even free jejunal transfer with omental cover may be employed.

Cancer of the lip and oral cavity

Due to the complications associated with irradiating the oral cavity and the availability of many flexible forms of reconstruction, surgery is now the primary treatment of choice in most cases. In many cases of recurrent disease it is also the chosen modality for similar reasons. The modern workhorse of oral cancer surgery is the radial forearm free flap, which can incorporate one or more paddles of thin pliable skin as well as bone if desired. However, for a primary jaw reconstruction, free fibular flap with multiple osteotomies is often preferred. The bulk of the tongue may be replaced by latissimus dorsi or rectus abdominis flaps. Oral cancer surgery, whether for early or late disease, should involve a multidisciplinary team including a head and neck surgeon, specialist prosthodontist, hygienist, dietitian, speech therapist, and specialist dental surgeon.

Saliva is important in moistening food to allow bolus formation, in maintaining oral flora that prevents development of dental caries, and in lubricating the oral mucosa to allow normal speech and swallowing. Xerostomia can be a severe and permanent complication of external beam radiation therapy. The sparing of at least one salivary gland can significantly reduce the sequelae of radiotherapy to the oral cavity. As a possible way of circumventing this problem, it has been proposed that translocation of at least one major salivary gland should be performed to an area outside the planned radiation field. There is some evidence that it does benefit patients,[33] and is certainly worthy of consideration. However, this is not always feasible and at present salivary substitutes is the mainstay of treatment. Surgery may have an increasing role in the future.

Cancer of the nasopharynx

Surgery has a limited role in recurrent disease. Occasionally if there is control of the primary, a neck dissection can be performed if there is persistent or recurrent neck disease. There are reports of using laser excision to debulk recurrence in the nasopharynx. Conventional surgery using combined craniofacial procedures via various approaches may have a greater chance of cure with less morbidity than re-irradiation in carefully selected patients,[34] though these are, in reality, rare.

It is common for patients with nasopharyngeal cancer to suffer from conductive hearing loss due to middle ear effusion. This may either be due to direct invasion of the Eustachian (auditory) tube, as a result of mass compression, or due to post-radiotherapy fibrosis. Grommet insertion can readily improve their hearing and eliminate the blocked ear sensation and, sometimes, pain.

Cancer of the oropharynx and hypopharynx

The role of palliative surgery in recurrent or advanced oropharyngeal cancer is limited to tracheostomy and laser debulking. The subject of combined glosso-laryngectomy with (non-functional) tongue reconstruction has excited controversy over many years. There are isolated reports of patients surviving 1 or 2 years with good quality of life after this very major procedure. However, in reality, the simultaneous loss of swallowing and speech combined with a very short life expectancy makes this an unreasonable option for most patients.

In contrast, recurrent and advanced hypopharyngeal cancer may necessitate total pharyngolaryngectomy. A degree of aided speech and reasonable swallowing may be expected after this procedure. Although it is a major undertaking for someone with limited life expectancy, it can achieve excellent symptom control. However, such major surgery risks equally major complications, including death from chest problems. Therefore, careful and realistic counselling with patient and relatives is required.

Cancer of the nose and sinus

About half of malignant sinus tumours are incurable. However, if surgical removal is not attempted, direct spread into mouth, eye, and brain may lead to an early death with blindness, deformity, bleeding, pain, trismus, and cerebrospinal fluid leak. Radiotherapy for large tumours in this area can also lead to severe complications, with damage to brainstem and eyes. As a result, the hand of the surgeon is often forced, even though positive margins are common. Such surgery should be the province of specialist teams, including cranio-facial and neurosurgical specialists. Epistaxis can persist, and the only way to stop it with minimum associated morbidity may be surgery. Sometimes, limited surgery may be used to decompress the orbit and preserve vision.

Young people with undifferentiated cancers of the maxillary sinus are a special problem. In patients with truly undifferentiated cancers, they are never cured by surgery and they should only be treated with radiotherapy. If surgery is required for palliative or curative intent, the surgeon must discuss and explain to the patient and relatives about the surgical implications. In order to treat the nose and sinus effectively, surgical intervention usually results in severe facial disfigurement. In such cases, prosthetics specialists must be involved early on prior to surgery to assist best planning and therefore rehabilitation.

Cancer of the skin and ear

Cancers of the middle ear are aggressive, often picked up late, and carry a relatively poor prognosis (35% disease-specific 5-year survival). Radical surgery is in the form of extended total petrosectomy with post-operative chemoradiotherapy. The head and ascending ramus of the mandible is resected with parotidectomy and pterygoid muscle resection as necessary. Dural resection and repair may be required. Occasionally extensive cancer involving the temporal lobe is treated by excision of the involved brain with a margin of normal tissue. The pinna and surrounding skin are sacrificed.

External auditory meatus cancer results are about 10% better than those of the middle ear and mastoid. Advanced cases may be treated with lateral or extended temporal bone resection as above, and reconstruction with a bulky free flap such as rectus abdominis can help. However, this procedure is effectively palliative due to the aggressive nature of this disease, and many patients do not leave hospital. Hence, detailed imaging and even preliminary surgery to determine the extent of the cancer are recommended before embarking on 'heroic' action. At a simpler level, surgery can remove necrotic or invaded bone, which may help alleviate pain. The resulting cavity can be used for drainage and inspection.

Cancer of the pinna often recurs, with extensive local infiltration and neck nodes. Prognosis is poor and, whilst multiple sequential resections often take place, the surgeon is always 'chasing' the disease. Nonetheless, such procedures do reduce fungation and pain.

Cancer of the major salivary glands

Cancer of the parotid gland is more common than those of the submandibular gland, though both are rare (about 500 per annum in the UK). The main surgical dilemmas in parotid cancer surgery revolve around preservation of the facial nerve. Some evidence suggests disease-free survival, though not overall prognosis, may improve if the facial nerve is resected in known cases of parotid cancer.[36] For established facial nerve paresis, lateral tarsorrhaphy and/or gold weight insertion in the upper eyelid improve eye closure. Static or dynamic facial reanimation is used in long-term cases, but is inappropriate in the palliative setting. Simple face-lifts or static slings may occasionally be used to improve appearance. Extensive surgery, including mandibular ramus excision and petrosectomy, is occasionally performed with palliative intent in very advanced cases.

Cancer of the thyroid and parathyroid glands

Thyroid cancers can be quite advanced at presentation or have recurrence in the neck or elsewhere and yet still have a reasonably good chance of a cure or longer survival compared with squamous cell carcinoma of the head and neck. Tracheal involvement is not uncommon. Invasive disease will require resection. A wedge resection of the trachea is performed for a localized disease. A more extensive disease will require a sleeve resection. In general, up to 4 cm of the trachea can be resected with primary anastomosis following suprahyoid release and mobilization of the trachea down to the carina. Newer technologies including tissue engineering may improve our ability to reconstruct tracheal resections in the future.

For thyroid lymphoma, the role of surgery is mainly in obtaining histological confirmation but also for removal of bulky disease. This has been shown to improve local control and survival. Sometimes, however, chemotherapy for locally advanced lymphomas may result in a tracheo-oesophageal fistula. This may require an endoscopically inserted oesophageal tube to prevent aspiration pneumonia.

The only useful surgery in anaplastic carcinoma is palliative. Isthmusectomy provides some material for histology and relief of local obstruction for a time. Tracheostomy is necessary in most cases to relieve impending airway obstruction from tumour and recurrent laryngeal nerve paralysis. If there is any doubt about the histological diagnosis, then a repeat biopsy is warranted as thyroid lymphoma can occasionally be mistaken for anaplastic cancer. Further care should involve the palliative care team.

Parathyroid carcinoma is rare. It occurs in about 1% of patients with primary hyperparathyroidism. Lymph node metastases occur in about 30% of cases. The treatment is by wide local excision including ipsilateral thyroid lobectomy and regional lymph nodes. There is little role for palliative surgery here as death is usually due to the metabolic consequences of gross hypercalcaemia.

Rare cancers

Lymphoid malignancy is treated with radiotherapy and chemotherapy, or a combination of both. Apart from the situations described for thyroid lymphoma above, and for obtaining tissue for staging and diagnosis, surgery has no role in palliation.

For bone sarcomas, palliation for recurrences is mainly non-surgical. However, with soft tissue sarcoma, e.g. adult-type soft-tissue sarcoma, surgery can be used for recurrences. Occasionally it is possible to resect an isolated lung metastasis and sometimes such patients become long-term survivors. In patients with rhabdomyosarcoma, radical surgery is occasionally indicated if there is residual disease following chemo-radiotherapy.

The primary site of mucosal malignant melanoma is usually in the nose or paranasal sinuses. Palliative surgery has little or no role in recurrences.

Paragangliomas are usually benign, but approximately 5% are malignant. They can produce distant metastases in bone and lung. Surgery is usually performed for lesions confined to the middle ear and mastoid. Advances in operative technique have now allowed more radical surgery to be done safely for lesions extending into the petrous temporal bone or with intracranial disease.

Kaposi's sarcoma is multifocal in nature, treated with radiotherapy and chemotherapy. Surgery is restricted to diagnosis and staging.

Conclusions

The word 'palliation' is still regarded as an acceptance of defeat by many surgeons engaged in an attempt to salvage advanced or recurrent cancer patients. For example, one surgical author argues that the patient and carers should be given the opportunity to consider surgical resection (with or without reconstruction) 'with the glimmer of hope for long-term survival and not automatically be forfeited to hospice and palliative care'.[27] However, is it really fair to offer a 'glimmer of hope', when the reality is palliative care in any case. The use of the term 'forfeited to...palliative care' also illustrates nicely the gulf in understanding of what palliative care means and can offer. Clearly, a considerable culture change is still required to make surgeons think appropriately about palliative care services.

Surgeons by definition are at their best when they are performing surgery. In most cases, the delineation between curative and palliative surgeries is clear. However, in other cases, the initial intention may be curative irrespective of the chances of success. These may eventually turn out to be overly optimistic and hence the intention becomes palliative in nature. However, it has become clear in the last few decades that surgery on its own has serious limitations, hence the need for a multidisciplinary approach involving head and neck specialist nurses, radiologists, head and neck surgeons, speech and swallow therapists, oncologists, and dietitians. The palliative specialist must now be included in this group to provide balance to decision making and to improve communication lines.

Surgery will remain an essential tool in palliative management in head and neck cancer patients for the foreseeable future. This is mainly due to the nature of advanced or recurrent head and neck cancer, which is usually locoregional. Surgery as palliation needs to be considered in the context of measurable palliation, patient co-morbidity, risk of complications, and quality of life before being undertaken. Despite the importance of surgery as a palliative tool in head and neck cancer, there have been no clinical trials in this area. These should now be designed as a collaboration between head and neck surgeons and palliative care teams, with minimization of surgical morbidity and of overall hospital stay as outcome measures. Likewise, at present, there is no set of guidelines on palliative surgery, with scant attention paid to it in national guidelines for head and neck cancer care in the UK. This too needs attention.

Surgical involvement in palliative care of the head and neck patient is a two-way process. Surgeons require a greater awareness of the principles of palliative care and, despite the present logistical problems, need to seek more help from local palliative care teams. Likewise, oncologists, palliative care physicians, and associated paramedical staff all need to be aware of those surgical options which exist for this, arguably the most unfortunate group of cancer patients.

Acknowledgements

We wish to express our gratitude to Mrs Elizabeth Bethan (MacMillan Specialist Head and Neck Cancer Nurse, North Bristol NHS Trust) and Mr Graham Porter (Consultant Head and Neck Surgeon, Southmead Hospital and St Michael's Hospital, Bristol) for their assistance during the embryonic stage of this chapter.

References

1 Wight, R., and The United Kingdom Association of Cancer Registries (2006). *DAHNO First Annual Report: key findings from the national head and neck cancer audit*, pp. 30–40. Leeds, NHS Health and Social Care Information Centre.

2 Sobin, L., and Wittekind, Ch. (2002). *TNM classification of malignant tumours*. John New Jersey, Wiley & Sons.

3 O'Sullivan, B., MacKillop, W., and Gilbert, R. (1994). Controversies in the management of laryngeal cancer: results of an international survey of patterns of care. *Radiother Oncol*, **31**, 23–32.

4 Short, S., Kaplan, J., Laramore, G., and Cummings, C. (1984). Shoulder pain and function after neck dissection with or without preservation of the spinal accessory nerve. *Am J Surg*, **148**, 478–482.

5 Hardin, M., VanDenmark, D., and Morris, H. (1990). Long-term speech results of cleft palate speakers with marginal velopharyngeal competence. *J Commun Disord*, **23**, 401–416.

6 McWilliams, B., Morris, H., and Shelton, R. (1994). *Cleft palate speech.* St Louis, Missouri, CV Mosby Company.

7 Nylen, B. (1961). Cleft palate speech. A surgical study including observations on velopharyngeal closure during connected speech, using synchronized cineradiography and sound spectrography. *Acta Radiol Suppl,* **203**, 1–124.

8 Blocksma, R. (1963). Correction of velopharyngeal insufficiency by silastic pharyngeal implant. *Plast Reconstruct Surg,* **31**, 268.

9 Lewy, R., Cole, R., and Wepman, J. (1965). Teflon injection in the correction of velopharyngeal insufficiency. *Ann Otol, Rhinol Laryngol,* **74**, 874.

10 Netterville, J., and Vrabec, J. (1994). Unilateral palatal adhesion for paralysis after high vagal injury. *Arch Otolaryngol Head Neck Surg,* **120**, 218–221.

11 Thomson, C., and Allison, R. (1997). The temporalis muscle flap in intraoral reconstruction. *Aust NZ J Surg,* **67**, 878–882.

12 Fan, K., Hopper, C., Speight, P., Buonaccorsi, G., and Brown, S. (1997). Photodynamic therapy using mTHPC for malignant disease in the oral cavity. *Int J Cancer,* **73**, 25–32.

13 Zeitels, S., Hillman, R., Desloge, R., and Bunting, G. (1999). Cricothyroid subluxation: a new innovation for enhancing the voice with laryngoplastic phonosurgery. *Ann Otol, Rhinol Laryngol,* **108**, 1126–1131.

14 Zeitels, S., Mauri, M., and Dailey, S. (2004). Adduction arytenopexy for vocal fold paralysis: indications and techniques. *J Laryngol Otol,* **118**, 508–516.

15 Mahieu, H., Norbart, T., and Snel, F. (1996). Laryngeal framework surgery for voice improvement. *Rev Laryngol Otol Rhinol,* **117**, 189–197.

16 Selz, P., and Santos, P. (1995). A useful tool for the Otolaryngologist–head and neck surgeon. *Arch Otolaryngol Head Neck Surg,* **121**, 1249–1252.

17 Mandal, A., Steel, A., Davidson, A., and Ashby, C. (2000). Day case percutaneous endoscopic gastrostomy: a viable proposition? *Postgrad Med J,* **76**, 157–159.

18 Paiva, M., Blackwell, K., Saxton, R., *et al.* (1998). Palliative laser therapy for recurrent head and neck cancer: a phase II clinical study. *Laryngoscope* **108**, 1277–1283.

19 Marks, J., Freeman, R., Lee, F., and Ogura, J. (1978). Pharyngeal wall cancer: analysis of treatment results, complications and patterns of failures. *Int J Radiat Oncol Biol, Phys,* **4**, 587–593.

20 Kluth, E., Jain, P., and Stutchell, R. (1987). A study of factors contributing to the development of osteonecrosis of the jaws. *J Prosthet Dent,* **58**, 78–82.

21 Marx, R. (1983). A new concept in the treatment of osteoradionecrosis. *J Oral Maxillofac Surg,* **41**, 351–357.

22 Withers, H., Peters, L., and Taylor, J. (1995). Late normal tissue sequela from radiation therapy for carcinoma of the tonsil: patterns of fractionation study of radiobiology. *Int J Radiat Oncol Biol, Phys,* **33**, 563–568.

23 Callahan, C. (2004). Facial disfigurement and sense of self in head and neck cancer. *Soc Work Health Care,* **40**, 73–87.

24 Wolfaardt, J., Sugar, A., and Wilkes, G. (2003). Advanced technology and the future of facial prosthetics in head and neck reconstruction. *Int J Oral Maxillofac Surg,* **32**, 121–123.

25 Goodwin, W.J., Jr (2000). Salvage surgery for patients with recurrent squamous cell carcinoma of the upper aerodigestive tract: when do the ends justify the means? *Laryngoscope,* **110**, 1–18.

26 Pitman, K., and Bradley, P. (2003). Management of the N3 neck. *Curr Opin Otolaryngol Head Neck Surg*, 11, 129–133.

27 Freeman, S. (2005). Advanced cervical metastasis involving the carotid artery. *Curr Opin Otolaryngol Head Neck Surg*, 13, 107–111.

28 Gavilan, J., Ferlito, A., Silver, C., Shaha, A., Martin, L., and Rinaldo, A. (2002). Status of carotid resection in head and neck cancer. *Acta Otolaryngol*, 122, 453–455.

29 Steiner, W., Vogt, P., Ambrosch, P., and Kron, M. (2004). Transoral carbon dioxide laser microsurgery for recurrent glottic carcinoma after radiotherapy. *Head Neck*, 26, 477–484.

30 Watkinson, J., Gaze, M., and Wilson, J. (2000). Tumour of the larynx. In Stell, P.M. and Maran, A.G.D. *Head and neck surgery*, pp. 233–274. Oxford, Butterworth Heinemann.

31 Gokhale, A., and Lavertu, P. (2001). Surgical salvage after chemoradiation of head and neck cancer complication and outcomes. *Curr Oncol Rep*, 3, 72–76.

32 Gluckman, J., Righi, P., Schuller, D., and Hamaker, R. (1994). Stomal recurrence following total laryngectomy. In Smee, R. and Bridger, G., eds. *Laryngeal cancer, Proceedings of the 2nd World Congress on Laryngeal Cancer*, pp. 621–624. Oxford, Elsevier.

33 Riegers, J., Seikaly, H., Jha, N., *et al.* (2005). Submandibular gland transfer for prevention of xerostomia after radiation therapy: swallow outcomes. *Arch Otolaryngol Head Neck Surg*, 131, 140–145.

34 Wei, W. (2000). Salvage surgery for recurrent primary nasopharyngeal carcinoma. *Crit Rev Oncol-Hematol*, 33, 91–98.

35 Calearo, C., Pastore, A., Storchi, O., and Polli, G. (1998). Parotid gland carcinoma: analysis of prognostic factors. *Ann Otol, Rhinol Laryngol*, 107, 969–973.

Chapter 3

The non-surgical management of advanced head and neck cancer

Frances Calman

Introduction

Head and neck cancer is the 12th most common cause of death from cancer in the UK but the seventh most common cause worldwide. More than half a million men and women in the world develop head and neck cancer each year and it accounts for approximately 2000 deaths per year in the UK.

In the UK, treatment is usually concentrated in large centres where expertise in all of the treatment and support modalities is concentrated. Once a patient returns home, however, he may find that his local support team only encounters a few patients with advanced head and neck cancer each year, and their experience in managing complex symptomatology is limited. Head and neck cancers tend to metastasize at a late stage so that locally recurrent disease is a cause of major morbidity especially as its anatomical situation in the body means that it frequently affects the ability to breathe, swallow, and speak.

There are five major head and neck cancer sites not including thyroid cancer. These are the oral cavity, the pharynx (further subdivided into the oropharynx, nasopharynx, and hypopharynx), the larynx, the paranasal sinuses, and the salivary glands. The pattern of lymphatic drainage differs for each site, and the prognosis worsens significantly if the disease extends further than the first echelon nodes and particularly if lower neck nodes are involved at presentation. Squamous carcinoma is the most common histological type at all sites except the nasopharynx and salivary glands.

Tobacco smoking and alcohol are the two most significant aetiological agents for most head and neck cancers, and the majority of patients are over the age of 60. Most patients are men, and with decreasing rates of cigarette consumption in the UK the incidence of head and neck cancer has fallen by almost 20% in the past 10 years, although the incidence in women is falling less swiftly, partly reflecting the fact that more women continue to smoke.

Many patients have significant co-morbidities associated with their lifestyle which make them poor candidates for radical treatment, and these factors may significantly affect treatment decisions. Alcoholism and alcohol-related diseases are common, and many patients suffer from relative malnutrition due to their poor diet. They are frequently isolated from family support and may live solitary lives in poor housing conditions, suspicious of intervention from well-meaning support and health care agencies. Their isolation may be further increased by treatment-associated morbidity (surgical mutilation, or loss of speech or the ability to swallow) or the effects of progressive disease (visible fungating wounds or severe neuralgic pain).

Results of treatment are excellent in early stage disease, and more than 80% of patients with T1 cancers of the head and neck are cured; however, the results of treatment of advanced disease are generally poor and all forms of treatment are associated with significant morbidity. The appalling distress caused by uncontrolled and progressive disease in the head and neck and the fact that tumours metastasize only late in the disease justifies radical and aggressive attempts to gain local control by surgery, radiotherapy, chemotherapy, or a combination of all treatment modalities. In the management of advanced disease where cure is infrequent, it is of the utmost importance that patients are aware of the full implications of treatment-related morbidity so that they can make the appropriate decisions between differing treatment modalities, and when fully informed patients will often accept a lower probability of cure in exchange for organ-preserving treatment.[1] Many patients find it difficult accessing information from written literature and frequently require repeated sessions of explanation and verbal information on a one-to-one basis with a health care worker whom they come to know and trust before coming to appropriate decisions regarding the treatment options available to them. Although curing the cancer is the major priority for almost all patients, it is essential that they understand the long-term morbidity of the treatments available and its impact on their quality of life. Explaining the challenges of living with a permanent gastrostomy, artificial speech, or major surgical disfigurement is difficult, although high-profile patients help to illustrate the problems[2] and many units use patient mentors to assist in the decision process. In advanced disease where cure rates by any modality are low, the patient has to understand that even very aggressive treatment with radical surgery and reconstruction followed by high-dose radiotherapy and concomitant chemotherapy may result in a cure rate of only 35% and that he may go through the trauma of complex multimodality treatment only to face untreatable recurrence within a year. The somewhat lesser morbidity of radical radiotherapy may result in a cure rate of 25% for the same disease, and this may be more acceptable to some patients.

The majority of head and neck cancers are squamous cancers

Smoking and alcohol are the most important aetiological factors

The majority of patients are over 60 years of age

Cure rates are low when the disease speads to lymph nodes

Choice of treatment modality

Where local control rates for differing treatments are the same, then the decision regarding the appropriate treatment modality rests on a comparison of the acute and long-term morbidity (or mortality) of the differing treatments.

In early laryngeal cancer, the probability of cure with radical radiotherapy is approximately 90–95%, and voice quality after treatment is good, but the treatment usually involves at least a 3 or 4 week course of daily treatment at a radiotherapy centre. All patients develop an acutely sore throat at the end of treatment which lasts approximately 3 weeks, and during that time nutrition may be difficult. Voice-conserving surgery (usually laser excision of the tumour) involves a single operation under general anaesthetic, two or three nights in hospital, a sore throat for about 7–10 days and, depending on the size of the tumour excised, an acceptable voice at the end of treatment. The local recurrence rates with this type of surgery are higher than with radiotherapy treatment and so up to 25% of patients subsequently require radiotherapy when they develop recurrent disease.

Local control of a moderately advanced tonsillar carcinoma with either radical radiotherapy or radical surgery and reconstruction is approximately 70%. In spite of excellent modern reconstructive techniques, there may be problems with speech and swallowing after surgery and if, because of close or positive margins or involved lymph nodes, the patient requires post-operative radiotherapy the functional results of surgery are severely compromised. Radical radiotherapy for tonsillar carcinoma may have significant acute morbidity but, in the long term, apart from a dry mouth, speech and swallowing are unaffected and there are no external marks of the treatment. The addition of concomitant chemotherapy adds to the acute morbidity of radiotherapy and there may be a requirement for enteral nutrition for up to 6 months, but again the prognosis for a return to normal swallowing is good.

Radiotherapy treatment

Radiotherapy is the most important non-surgical treatment for head and neck cancer, and its organ-preserving capabilities make it an attractive alternative to surgery. In advanced disease, however, cure rates are low with radiotherapy alone, and mutimodal treatment with combinations of radiotherapy, chemotherapy, surgery, and possibly biological agents is necessary to improve cure rates.

Radiotherapy is given as a course of daily treatments usually lasting 4–6 weeks. Treatment accuracy is of the utmost importance, with high doses of radiation delivered to small volumes of tissue which are frequently in close proximity to vital and radiosensitive structures such as the eye, the spinal cord, and the brainstem. Patients are treated in an immobilizing shell (Fig. 3.1) and the treatment volume is frequently defined using computed tomography (CT) imaging in order to maximize the accuracy of treatment. Treatment may be given in two or three phases with gradually reducing volumes to minimize long-term side effects of treatment, reduce doses to critical structures, and deliver higher doses to areas of gross disease rather than those areas with microscopic or subclinical disease (see Figs 3.2–3.4).

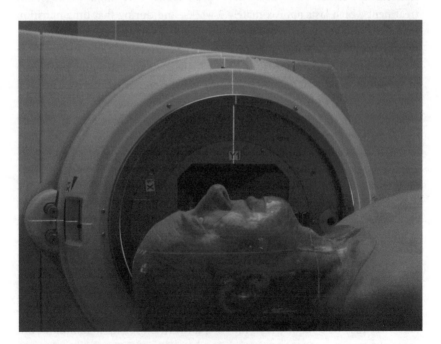

Fig. 3.1 A patient having treatment in an immobilization shell.

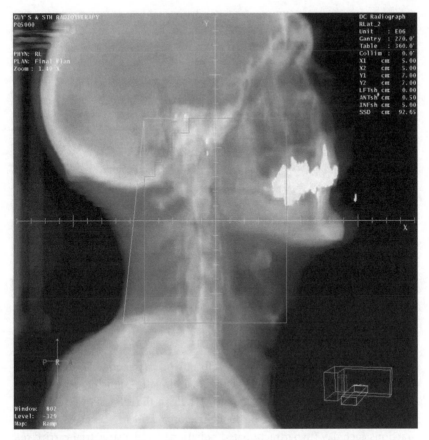

Fig. 3.2 Volume for phase I treatment of tonsillar carcinoma outlined on a digitally reconstructed radiograph.

Fractionation

Radiotherapy treatment is given in divided doses (fractions) each day in order to minimize the long-term side effects of treatment. Squamous carcinoma is a rapidly proliferating tumour, and undue prolongation of treatment time can allow regrowth of the cancer between fractions. For this reason the overall treatment time is kept as short as possible, and preferably between 4 and 6 weeks.

Randomized trials carried out in Denmark showed that the same dose of radiation given in 5 weeks instead of 6 weeks had a significantly higher local control rate and therefore higher laryngeal preservation.[3] Further reduction of overall time to 4 weeks, however, caused increased severe complications[4] and necessitated a reduction in total dose.

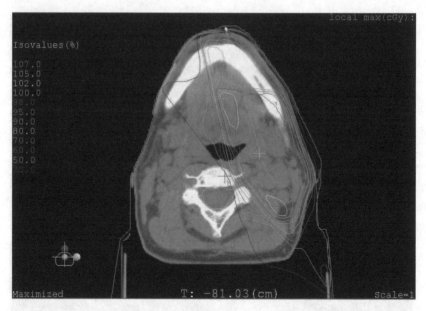

Fig. 3.3 CT slice showing the radiation isodoses to treat a localized volume including the left tonsil and involved lymph nodes.

Normal tissue repair takes place rapidly after each fraction of radiation, and the majority of repair has taken place within 4 h, allowing radiotherapy treatments to be given more frequently. Trials in the USA showed that local control was improved if part of the course of treatment was given with two fractions each day (hyperfractionated radiation),[5] and a large trial carried out in the UK demonstrated that a lower dose of radiation given in three fractions each day every day for 12 consecutive days [continuous hyperfractionated accelerated radiation treatment (CHART)] had equivalent effects in terms of local control and complications as a higher dose given in conventional frac-tionation over 6 weeks.[6] The side effects of this more concentrated form of treatment are at least as severe as more prolonged courses of treatment, and this more intense way of delivering treatment has not been widely adopted, largely because of logistic problems associated with the need to treat patients outside of the normal working day and at weekends.

Hypoxia

All clinically detectable squamous cancers have hypoxic regions which are more resistant to radiation and therefore reduce the probability of local control. Maintaining the haemoglobin level above 12 g/dl is a relatively simple and effective way of minimizing hypoxia. In the past, hyperbaric oxygen was

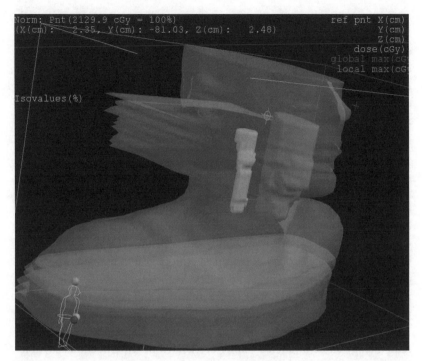

Fig. 3.4 Three-dimensional reconstruction of the patient showing the treatment volume and the spinal cord.

tried in an effort to overcome hypoxia, but was difficult to administer and the majority of clinical trials failed to show advantage for hyperbaric oxygen in head and neck cancer. Most attempts at pharmacological sensitization of hypoxic cells have been ineffective; however, trials of the imidazole drug nimorazole (one of a group of drugs including antifungal agents miconazole and fluconazole) showed significant benefit.[3] Nimorazole is given orally but causes nausea in about a third of patients, which limits its use. It is not available in the UK, but small-scale trials have been carried out using supplies of the drug imported from Denmark where it is routinely used in the treatment of patients with head and neck cancer. There are trials currently underway of the new hypoxic cell sensitizer tirapazamine which appears to be a highly active agent.

Systemic chemotherapy

Although response rates to chemotherapy in untreated squamous cancers of the head and neck are fairly high, of the order of 60–70%, the median duration of response is short, and generally only a few months, making primary treatment with chemotherapy inappropriate. In recurrent or metastatic disease, response rates to chemotherapy in previously unirradiated tissue are significantly higher than in previously irradiated tissue; however, the median duration of response is of the order of 3–6 months, making chemotherapy unhelpful as a sole treatment modality apart from short-term palliation in the otherwise fit patient. The most active agents are cisplatin, carboplatin, and infusional 5-fluorouracil, although newer cytotoxics such as the taxanes and capecitabine are active and may produce equivalent or improved response rates without higher toxicity.

Following the publication of a large meta-analysis,[7] the use of chemotherapy given synchronously with radiotherapy has become widespread practice in advanced disease. This gives a benefit of approximately 5–10% in local control and somewhat lower rates of improvement in survival when compared with conventional radiotherapy alone. Although the local control rates are improved, the acute toxicity of treatment with radical radiotherapy and concomitant chemotherapy is increased and patients require considerable support in symptom control of the more severe mucositis and also a more prolonged period of nutritional support before normal swallowing may be established.

No trials have been done comparing concomitant chemo-radiotherapy with radiotherapy alone in altered (either accelerated or hyperfractionated) fractionation, and it is unproven whether the addition of chemotherapy to radiotherapy confers additional benefit to that obtained with optimal altered fractionation. At present the most common agent used synchronously with radiotherapy is cisplatin which has demonstrated activity against squamous carcinoma but also activity as a radiosensitizer. It is normally administered as an infusion every 7–21 days. In some centres this can be administered as an out-patient treatment but may involve an overnight stay. The drug is excreted through the kidneys, and renal function has to be reasonably good to allow the drug to be eliminated from the body. It is otherwise well tolerated, the main side effect being nausea which is usually well controlled with modern antiemetic regimens.

Biological agents

Many head and neck cancers overexpress epidermal growth factor receptors and this may be one of the causes of cells proliferating very rapidly in the cancer process. Administering a monoclonal antibody to epidermal growth factor receptors, such as cetuximab, has limited activity on its own in head and neck cancer, but recent studies have shown that benefit is gained from administering it at the same time as radiation.[8] It also appears to have activity when given with platinum-based chemotherapy in patients who have relapsed after having cisplatin chemotherapy or who have become resistant to platinum chemotherapy. The order of benefit (~10%) when given with radiotherapy is approximately the same as that obtained by administering concomitant chemotherapy, and there is now considerable interest in combining it with chemotherapy as well as radiotherapy in the treatment of advanced head and neck cancer. The most serious complications of cetuximab treatment are allergic or anaphylactic reactions. The majority of patients develop an acneiform rash and it is suggested that the rash may be a marker of activity as those patients with a more severe rash appear to respond better to treatment.

Surgery and radiotherapy are the main treatment modalities

Surgery or radiotherapy alone may be indicated in early stage disease with equally good results

Advanced disease frequently requires combined modality treatment using surgery, radiotherapy, and chemotherapy

The addition of biological agents may improve treatment results further

---

Acute side effects of radiotherapy

Mucositis

The most common acute side effect of treatment is mucositis within the treated area. The epithelial surface of the mouth and upper airways is continuously repaired and replaced with cells rising from the bases of crypts and mucous glands to populate the layers of the intact epithelium; these cells then mature and rise to the surface of the epithelium before being shed from the surface. Radiotherapy treatment damages the immature cells in the basement layers of the glands so that there are no new cells to replace those shed from the surface of the epithelium, and ulceration occurs. Exudate which forms on the surface of the denuded mucosa is termed a 'membrane'. As the radiation damage continues, the basement layers containing nerve endings and blood vessels are exposed causing severe pain and bleeding. This process becomes apparent during the second or third week of treatment and continues until approximately 2–3 weeks after the end of the course of treatment when it heals completely.

Loss of taste

Where the treatment volume includes the taste buds of the tongue or oral cavity, taste is affected at an early stage in the course of treatment and recovers very slowly after the completion of radiotherapy, usually returning to normal by 6 months after completion of treatment in all but those patients who have received the maximum dose of radiation to the posterior third of the tongue.

Dryness

Dryness of the mouth is the most disabling long-term side effect of radiotherapy for advanced head and neck cancer. The major salivary glands are commonly included in the treatment volume because of their close proximity either to the primary tumour or to node-bearing regions and, although some function may slowly return following treatment, it rarely returns to normal and persistent dryness significantly affects the quality of life in treated patients. Many patients are forced to make long-term dietary modifications in order to cope with the dryness; most return to a fairly normal diet but avoid very dry or crumbly food such as pastry, cakes, or biscuits, and take all of their food with plenty of moisture. A small number never return to normal eating and require a liquidized diet for the rest of their lives.

Reducing the morbidity of treatment

Conformal radiotherapy

Radiotherapy treatment is conventionally delivered using a small number of fixed fields to encompass known disease and areas at high risk of subclinical involvement. The shape of these fields may be altered using customized lead to shield tissue which does not need to be treated, and the position of this lead can be very accurately calculated using CT scans. In this way, the treatment volume can be tailored with great precision but the shape of the volume treated must always be convex, as in a sphere, or cylinder, or ellipsoid shape.

IMRT

Intensity-modulated radiotherapy (IMRT) is increasingly used in an attempt to reduce the morbidity of radiotherapy for head and neck cancer. This involves highly sophisticated treatment planning to exclude critical organs such as salivary glands and spinal cord from the high-dose treatment volume with the aim of increasing the dose delivered to the tumour whilst reducing the long-term side effects of treatment. Up to seven or nine fields may be used and, during the treatment, metal shielding leaves are electronically moved in and out of the radiation beam to allow higher doses of radiation to be given to some parts of the field rather than others. The treatment volumes can be sculpted to treat concave shapes such as when a tumour curves round the spinal cord and paraspinal tissues. Even greater accuracy of immobilization is required than for conventional or conformal radiotherapy, and the treatment time each day is greatly increased because more numerous treatment fields are used in order to shape the beam to avoid critical organs and reduce the long-term side effects of treatment. The initial results of this form of treatment suggest that local control is not compromised by greater use of shielding of normal structures, and objective measures of resting and stimulated salivary flow confirm that the planning techniques are successful in achieving the aims of sparing normal tissue. Because of the necessarily large volumes treated in advanced head and neck cancer, it may not be possible to reduce the side effects of treatment significantly enough to affect quality of life positively in all patients; however, IMRT may also allow higher doses to be delivered to tumour-bearing areas and therefore improve local control.

Radioprotectors

Radioprotectors have been used in an attempt to minimize the long-term side effects of treatment, especially the problems of dry mouth. They are absorbed into normal tissues and bring about chemical changes which make the cells less likely to be damaged by radiation. At present it is not certain that they do not also protect the cancer and their use is still the subject of clinical trials. The most widely used radioprotector is amifostine, which is given as an intravenous infusion each day prior to treatment. The main side effect is nausea, and this in association with the need for a daily intravenous infusion makes it unpopular with a group of patients who seek as little contact with hospitals and as little intervention as possible.

Laryngeal cancer

Laryngeal cancer affects 2300 persons per year in the UK, of whom 80% are men and 70% are over the age of 60 years. Cure rates have not changed greatly over the past 30 years, and approximately 60% of patients are cured of their disease, reflecting the fact that the majority of patients present with early stage disease; however, it is the most common cause of death from head and neck cancer in the UK.

Patients with cancer of the vocal cords usually present with a hoarse voice and, when patients present with advanced disease, there has frequently been a delay in presentation or diagnosis. Nodal involvement only occurs when the primary cancer is advanced. Cancer of the supraglottic larynx may be more insidious in onset and therefore more difficult to diagnose at an early and curable stage. Although it only causes hoarseness when more advanced, patients often complain of discomfort in the throat or a change in voice. The natural history of supraglottic carcinoma is to metastasize to lymph nodes earlier, and cure rates are less good than for glottic cancer. Pain is rarely a problem in laryngeal cancer except in the case of patients with supraglottic cancer who may develop persistent, and sometimes severe, neuropathic pain radiating to the ear as a result of parapharyngeal extension of disease or perineural invasion. This may occur even in apparently early stage disease and is associated with a poorer outcome.

Where the presenting tumour invades the laryngeal cartilage or is so bulky as to obstruct the airway, cure rates with radiotherapy alone are poor. Otherwise healthy patients are usually advised to have primary surgery (total laryngectomy and ipsilateral neck dissection) followed by radiotherapy if there are adverse features such as extralaryngeal spread of disease, positive resection margins, nodal extracapsular spread, or multiple involved nodes. Many patients undergo voice reconstruction with the insertion of speaking valves at the time of primary surgery or after completion of post-operative radiotherapy; however, about 20% of patients fail to achieve any voice after surgery even with modern reconstruction. For a significant proportion of patients, a laryngectomy is not acceptable, and for those patients concomitant chemo-radiotherapy can offer cure rates of up to 25% in advanced disease. Where there are clinically involved lymph nodes, the cure rate is significantly lower and future advances in treatment may lie in biological agents such as epidermal growth factor receptor antibodies.

Laryngeal cancer

Laryngeal cancer is the most common head and neck cancer in the UK

Early laryngeal cancer is highly curable

Survival is poor if lymph nodes are involved

20% of patients never achieve a voice after radical sugery

Oral and oropharyngeal cancer

Oral and oropharyngeal cancer together form the seventh most common cancers in the EU and the 14th most common cause of death from cancer. They are very closely related to tobacco and alcohol intake, and the incidence rises across Europe from 9.3 cases per 100 000 in the UK to 40 per 100 000 in Hungary. The death rates are variable, reflecting co-morbidities and stage at presentation; in the UK, the death rate from oral cancer is 4.2 per 100 000 but rises to 25.8 per 100 000 in Hungary which also has the highest death rate from lung cancer in Europe. Although the incidence of oral cancer in France is 46 per 100 000, the death rate in France is 15.9 per 100 000, reflecting public awareness of the disease and earlier presentation as well as expertise in specialist treatment. The incidence rate rises with age and is approximately twice as common in men as in women. Globally the highest incidence of oral cancer is in Sri Lanka and the Indian subcontinent, where it accounts for almost a third of new cases of cancer in men, compared with approximately 2% in the UK. This is due to the presence of susceptible genes for oral submucous fibrosis in the population and high rates of betel nut and tobacco chewing, as well as cigarette smoking and alcohol intake. In the UK, the death rates have not altered over the past 30 years, but the incidence has shown disturbing trends; the rates of oral cancer in older men are falling significantly but in men between the ages of 40 and 60 the incidence has almost doubled. Oral cancer rates in Scotland are much higher than elsewhere in the UK, reflecting high levels of alcohol intake and smoking. Recent public awareness campaigns hopefully will encourage patients to present earlier, but this is not a patient population which regularly visits dentists or doctors and it is difficult to target the high-risk groups for this disease.

Surgical treatment of advanced cancer of the oral cavity and oropharynx is mutilating and although reconstructive techniques have improved greatly with the advance of free-flap microvascular surgery, the functional results of surgery are greatly reduced when post-operative radiotherapy is added in order to improve local control. Many patients with advanced oral and oro-pharyngeal cancer present with significant nutritional impairment due to both lifestyle and the disease, and are poor candidates for radical surgery and post-operative radiotherapy. Whether treated with radical radiotherapy and concomitant chemotherapy or radical surgery and post-operative chemo-radiotherapy, the majority of patients require enteral feeding support throughout their management, but the probability of a return to normal speech and swallowing is greater after non-surgical treatment than after surgery alone or surgery and post-operative radiotherapy. The treatment decisions in this group of patients demand close collaboration between specialists in all treatment modalities, including clinical nurse specialists, speech and language therapists, and nutritional therapists, if the appropriate decisions regarding definitive treatment are to be made, and if the patients is to be allowed to make informed decisions regarding the treatment options.

Although the only curative treatment option in advanced disease may be surgery and post-operative chemo-radiotherapy, the patient has to understand that the chance of achieving cure may be less than 15% in some situations and that the chances of surviving for 1 year after treatment if it is unsuccessful are small. Although cure may not be possible, many patients can live independent and relatively normal lives after radiotherapy, and the evidence shows that patients live as long or longer after radiotherapy as after unsuccessful surgery. The period of rehabilitation after major oral surgery is long and arduous, and patients require good family and social support networks to survive.

Oral cancer

- ◆ Oral cancer accounts for a third of all new cases of cancer in Sri Lanka and the Indian sub-continent
- ◆ The main aetiological factors are tobacco and alcohol
- ◆ Pain is uncommon and patients frequently present with advanced disease

Cancer of the nasopharynx and paranasal sinuses

Carcinoma of the nasopharynx occurs most commonly in Eastern Asia and Eastern Africa where the undifferentiated type of histology is seen, associated with Epstein–Barr virus (EBV) infection. The primary tumour is often un-detected at an early stage, and patients present with the symptoms of advanced disease such as cranial nerve palsies or enlarging lymph nodes in the posterior triangle of the neck. The disease is uncommon in the UK and the early symptoms of disease are often unrecognized; any Chinese or East African presenting in the middle decades of life with nasal stuffiness or blood-stained nasal discharge, deafness due to a middle ear effusion, or persistent headache at the vertex should be considered to have a nasopharyngeal cancer until proved otherwise.

The diagnosis may be obvious on examination of the nasopharynx, but in some patients the primary tumour may not cause mucosal ulceration, and biopsies of the walls and roof of the nasopharynx may be required to make the diagnosis.

The treatment is radical radiotherapy given with concomitant chemother-apy. There is a high incidence of lymph node involvement even in the earliest stages of disease, and the primary tumour is treated in continuity with all of the lymph node-bearing areas above the clavicle even in stage I disease. In undifferentiated nasopharyngeal cancer, local control of disease is obtained in more than 75% of patients, but half develop distant metastases (commonly bone, liver, or lung) within 5 years. Trials are currently under way in Canada, Singapore, and Hong Kong to determine whether or not the addition of adjuvant chemotherapy after radical chemo-radiotherapy will reduce the rate of distant metastases.

In the UK, nasopharyngeal carcinoma is uncommon and is usually squamous carcinoma type, often presenting insidiously in the elderly. Lymph node metastases are uncommon and the tumour is frequently locally advanced, with destruction of the base of the skull and cranial nerve palsies at diagnosis. If patients are fit enough, the treatment is as for undifferentiated nasopharyngeal cancer but local control is less good and the prognosis is often poor, with small numbers of patients surviving more than a year after diagnosis.

Cancer of the paranasal sinuses is not associated with the usual aetiological factors associated with head and neck cancer, and generally the cause is unknown. Although relatively uncommon, it causes great distress and morbidity. The presenting symptoms of headache and nasal discharge are vague and often misdiagnosed until the cancer becomes more advanced, causing visual disturbance, neurological abnormalities, or facial swelling. The treatment is usually by a combination of surgery, which is often mutilating, followed by high-dose radiotherapy.

Cancer of the nasopharynx and paranasal sinuses

- Nasopharyngeal cancer is most common in China and South-East Asia
- Local control in nasopharyngeal cancer is greater than 70% with chemo-radiotherapy, but half of those die of metastases
- Cancer of the para-nasal sinuses is rare, and treatment requires both radical surgery and high-dose radiotherapy

Treatment of metastatic and recurrent disease

More than 70% of patients who die of advanced head and neck cancer die of locally recurrent disease, and in the majority of patients the recurrence declares itself within 2 years of completing radical treatment.

Surgical salvage

Salvage surgery is the best option for patients with recurrent cancer of the upper aerodigestive tract, with reported 5-year survival rates of 35–40%,[9] being highest when there is localized laryngeal relapse and lowest in relapse in the hypopharynx or the base of the tongue, or in neck nodes after definitive radiotherapy. Surgical salvage of relapse in the nasopharynx is rare and practised in only a few specialist centres in the world. Assessment of suitability for salvage surgery for recurrent head and neck cancer includes a detailed assessment of the general physical and psychological health of the patient as well as cancer-related factors to determine whether or not the cancer is resectable. Extensive resection of a locally advanced recurrent cancer and subsequent reconstruction involves lengthy and difficult surgery and a long period of rehabilitation afterwards. Salvage surgery is only possible in about 50% of patients who recur.

Increasingly, patients with advanced disease are treated with concomitant chemo-radiotherapy and, although the salvage rates after combined modality treatment are similar to those after radiotherapy alone, the complication rate following surgery is significantly higher in terms of reconstructive flap failure and fistula formation,[10] which has to be taken into account when counselling patients about the risks of surgery.

The cost to the patient of salvage surgery is high in terms of both acute and long-term morbidity and permanent disability. Where the probability of successful salvage is likely to be low, the best approach to recurrent disease for many patients and their families may be honest and compassionate discussion of the limited treatment options, and referral to an experienced palliative care team for symptom control and supportive care.

Salvage surgery

Surgical treatment after relapse is possible in fewer than 50% of patients

3-year survival after salvage surgery is less than 40%

The acute morbidity and mortality of salvage surgery is increased in heavily pre-treated patients

Palliative chemotherapy

Patients with advanced head and neck cancer frequently have multiple co-morbidities, making them poor candidates for intensive chemotherapy treatment. The drugs with the highest response rates are 5-fluorouracil given as a 4 or 5 day continuous infusion, and cisplatin, requiring a week in hospital every 3 or 4 weeks. Response rates in previously irradiated tissue are poor and usually less than 20%, although response rates in unirradiated tissue such as lung metastases may be higher. The median duration of response is short, around 4 months, making this a poor option for patients when quality of life measured without symptoms of disease or side effects of treatment may be only a few weeks.

The recent availability of oral forms of 5-fluorouracil may make it possible to reduce the time of in-patient stay, making the treatment more attractive to patients; however, the drug is currently not licensed for this use and treatment has to be within research trial protocols. The addition of Docetaxel appears to improve response rates in previously treated patients, but there are no randomized trials of different palliative agents[11] and in particular very few quality of life data for palliative chemotherapy.

Palliative chemotherapy

* The most active chemotherapy drugs are cisplatin and 5-fluorouracil
* Taxanes are active in recurrent head and neck cancer
* Response rates in disease recurring in previously irradiated tissue are less than 20%
* Median duration of response is 4–6 months

Re-irradiation

Radical re-treatment with radiotherapy has long been recognized as a treatment option for selected patients with recurrent head and neck cancer, but the morbidity of treatment is high and, when active cytotoxic agents became available in the 1970s, this treatment was abandoned in the hope that chemotherapy treatment would bring about good palliation without the risks and complications of further radiotherapy. That hope has not been achieved and there is now a re-evaluation of the role of radical re-irradiation in recurrent disease. We have a better understanding of the radiobiology of repair; modern imaging techniques and better treatment localization allow us to define our treatment volumes more accurately to reduce further damage. The best results are obtained where the volume of recurrent disease is small and the time interval between primary treatment and recurrence is more than 2 years. Full radical doses are required to control recurrent cancer, and almost all patients experience severe fibrosis in the irradiated field and trismus if the temporo-mandibular region is included. There is a significant risk of osteoradionecrosis, uncontrollable haemorrhage due to telangiectasia, and permanent nerve damage if significant neural tissue is included in the irradiated field. The risk of severe morbidity or mortality from re-treatment is approximately 20% and the probability of successful local control in reported series is between 20 and 35% at 5 years after re-irradiation in this selected group of patients.[12] This treatment modality should be considered in all patients who relapse locally more than 18 months after their primary radiotherapy.

Challenges for the future

It has been estimated that the incidence of this group of diseases would fall by at least 80% if smoking tobacco and drinking alcohol were abolished. A further small group of patients have virally related disease [either EBV or human papillomavirus (HPV)] which could be prevented by appropriate vaccines. In the Indian subcontinent, the additional abolition of betel-nut or pan chewing would further dramatically reduce the incidence of buccal carcinoma. Public education to ensure that patients present early with localized disease would also drastically reduce the incidence of recurrent and incurable disease. These diseases, however, affect a vulnerable group of people whose locus of self-control is often low and who are not easily able to give up smoking and alcohol. Until the incidence of these cancers can be reduced, they will continue to require the most complex treatment, support, and symptom control both at presentation and in the face of recurrent and incurable disease which will challenge all groups of workers associated with the management of head and neck cancer.

Case study

G.T. was a 53 year-old man who presented in March 2002 with a 3–4 month history of a painless enlarging lump, which measured 3 cm in diameter in the right side of the neck. He was an engaging articulate man with a somewhat 'alternative' lifestyle. He lived alone although he had a circle of close and supportive friends and was not in regular employment. His one daughter had died 10 years previously of new variant Jacob–Creutzfeld disease, and he had no contact with her mother. He smoked marijuana socially and had smoked cigarettes regularly in the past. He enjoyed a glass of wine but had never been a heavy drinker. His general health was excellent and he was a keen cyclist, regularly cycling the 15 miles from his home to the hospital to keep his appointments.

Fine needle aspiration cytology of the neck lump showed squamous carcinoma cells, and a subsequent examination under anaesthetic revealed a 2 cm mass in the right lateral base of the tongue. He underwent a right-sided neck dissection followed by 6 weeks of radiotherapy to the tongue base and both sides of the neck with weekly cisplatin chemotherapy during the radiotherapy. He tolerated the treatment extremely well, maintaining his nutrition in spite of the mucositis and cycling to the hospital for his treatment. At the end of treatment. there was no evidence of residual disease in his neck or oropharynx.

One year after completing his radiotherapy, he began to complain of neuralgic pain in the right side of the face and occasional difficulty in swallowing so that he felt as though he had to swallow twice. Cross-sectional imaging showed only thickening in the tissues in the right side of the neck in keeping with his previous radiotherapy, and examination under anaesthetic and biopsies of the base of the tongue revealed no sign of recurrent malignancy. His pain persisted and increased. He took regular co-codamol but refused opioids, and eventually found the most relief from 2% cocaine mouthwash, which we usually prescribe for the relief of pain in acute mucositis at the end of radiotherapy. A positron emision tomography (PET) scan showed greatly increased uptake in the base of the tongue and in the right side of the neck, but further biopsies failed to confirm malignancy. By this stage, his pain was severe and we made a diagnosis of recurrent malignancy in spite of the negative biopsies.

Nine months after the onset of his pain, there was obvious induration and thickening in the upper right neck and he had a series of episodes of brisk bleeding from the back of the mouth. We discussed the treatment options with him, namely salvage surgery or best supportive care. Salvage surgery would have involved a total glossectomy, probably a total laryngectomy, and reconstruction. Both speech and swallowing would probably have been impossible after the surgery although he might have managed to swallow some liquids. The probability of cure would have been less than 25% and the probability of dying from complications of the procedure was at least 10% in view of his previous surgery and radiotherapy. He decided against surgery. Had he expressed a wish to attempt surgery we would have made further attempts to obtain histological confirmation of recurrence before proceeding, but as he did not wish to pursue that route there was no compelling need to seek histological confirmation of the disease process.

In February 2004, he agreed to a trial of chemotherapy using cisplatin and 5-flourouracil. He hated the week's admission for each course of treatment, which restricted his activity, and he intensely disliked the communal lifestyle in the ward with six beds together and shared bathrooms. We had a long discussion regarding his resuscitation status and he asked some very direct questions, including what I thought might be the mode of his death and whether there was a chance that he might bleed to death. He did not want any attempts at resuscitation in case of cardio-pulmonary arrest, recognizing that although he was leading a fairly normal life at this stage, he had a progressive and incurable illness.

At the end of three courses of chemotherapy his symptoms were no better and we agreed that further chemotherapy would not be appropriate. His pain slowly increased and the movement of his tongue became more restricted, leading to increasing difficulties with both speech and swallowing. His medication was adjusted and he agreed to a trial of oral morphine sulfate, which he found helpful although he remained reluctant to increase the dose because of drowsiness. He did not tolerate tricyclic antidepressants but did take a modest dose of gabapentin which he also restricted because of drowsiness. As his difficulty swallowing increased, he struggled more and more to maintain his weight but refused to consider a gastrostomy. The reasons for this were complex but included issues around his daughter's long and painful death. Dysphagia had been an early feature of her illness and although he recognized that at first it had kept her alive, he also felt that it had prolonged her suffering. By this stage, there was obvious disease in the right upper neck and submandibular region which was bleeding and about to fungate. In January 2005, he agreed to further palliative radiotherapy in an attempt to stop further bleeding, but after only one of a planned five treatments he developed a fistula between the floor of his mouth and his neck. This further increased his difficulties in swallowing and added a moist discharging wound to his problems. Eventually when he had lost more than 20% of his body weight and was spending more than 4 h each day trying to get nourishment down, he reluctantly agreed to have a percutaneous gastrostomy inserted. He had spent his savings on a boat and his great wish was to sail round the British Isles but he found that he was too weak to do any sailing. He hoped that improving his nutrition would give him the strength to sail again. Stopping oral intake made the fistula immediately easier to manage and he began to gain a small amount of weight.

The fistula slowly enlarged and was very difficult to treat. It was highly exudative and also in a position under his jaw where dressings were difficult to maintain. He felt strangled by most bandages and attempts to keep dressings in place lasted only a few hours. When I last saw him early in September 2005, his speech was almost unintelligible and there was a loud sucking noise through the fistula, which had no dressing over it. He insisted on showing me the inside of the fistula with a mirror as he felt that there were some form of parasites with tubular suckers living in it; I had to tell him that even with a bright light and a good view of the fistula I could see nothing but the necrotic walls of the fistula covered with exudate. He also showed me some photographs taken a few weeks earlier of him sitting on his boat which he still hoped to be able to sail one day.

He was in regular contact with the local palliative care team but maintained largely social contact with them, preferring to control his own medication and dressings with minimal input from any outside agencies. He remained at home, getting weaker and thinner, and then one evening shortly after I had seen him, he had a large and brisk bleed from the back of his mouth whilst alone at home. He was unable to use the telephone and too weak to get to the door to summon help from neighbours. By chance, his District Nurse texted him to check that he was all right and he managed one word in reply: 'Help'. He was admitted to the hospice as an emergency having refused hospital admission and was cared for there for 4 weeks before his death from bronchopneumonia at the end of September 2005. Whilst an in-patient, he allowed his opioids to be titrated gradually to improve his pain control and he was more compliant with other medications such as gabapentin than he had been at home. He had a further very large haemorrhage in the hospice, but again survived it and remained lucid almost to the last, communicating in copious pages of hand-writing. In one of his last 'conversations' with his palliative care consultant he talked about 'The curse of hope'.

References

1 McNeil, B.J., Weichselbaum, R., and Pauker, S.G. (1981). Speech and survival: tradeoffs between quality and quantity of life in laryngeal cancer. *N Engl J Med*, **305**, 982–987.

2 Diamond, J. (2004). *Because cowards get cancer too*. London, Vermilion Books.

3 Overgaard, J., Hansen, H.S., Specht, L., *et al.* (2003). Five compared with six fractions per week of conventional radiotherapy of squamous cell carcinoma of head and neck: DAHANCA 6 and 7 randomised controlled trial. *Lancet*, **362**, 933–940.

4 Maciejewski, B., Skladowski, K., Pilecki, B., *et al.* (1996). Randomized clinical trial on accelerated 7 days per week fractionation in radiotherapy for head and neck cancer. Preliminary report on acute toxicity. *Radiother Oncol*, **40**, 137–145.

5 Fu, K.K., Pajak, T.F., Trotti, T.A., *et al.* (2000). A Radiation Therapy Oncology Group (RTOG) phase III randomised study to compare hyper fractionation and two variants of accelerated fractionation to standard fractionation radiotherapy for head and neck squamous cell carcinomas: first report of RTOG 9003. *Int J Radiat Oncol Biol Phys*, **48**, 7–16.

6. Dische, S., Saunders, M., Barrett, A., Harvey, A., Gibson, D., and Parmar, M. (1997). A randomised multicenter trial of CHART versus conventional radiotherapy in head and neck cancer. *Radiother Oncol*, **44**, 123–136.

7 Pignon, J.P., Bourhis, J., Domenge, C., and Designe, L. (2000). Chemotherapy added to loco regional treatment for head and neck squamous-cell carcinoma: three meta-analyses of updated individual data. MACH-NC Collaborative Group. Meta-Analysis of Chemotherapy on Head and Neck Cancer. *Lancet*, **3 55**, 949–955.

8 Bonner, J., Harari, P.M., and Giralt, J.L. (2004). Cetuximab prolongs survival in patients with locally advanced squamous cell carcinoma of the head and neck; a phase III study of high dose radiation therapy with or without cetuximab. *Proc Am Soc Clin Oncol* (abstract). 5507.

9 Goodwin, W.J., Jr (2000). Salvage surgery for patients with recurrent squamous cell cancer of the upper aero digestive tract: when do the ends justify the means? *Laryngoscope*, **110** Suppl 93, 1–18.

10 Weber, R.S., Berkey, B.A., Forestiere, A., *et al.* (2003). Outcome of salvage total laryngectomy following organ preservation therapy: the Radiation Oncology Group trial 91–11. *Arch Otolaryngol Head Neck Surg*, **129**, 44–49.

11 Pignon, J.P., Syz, N., Posner, M., *et al.* (2004). Adjusting for patient selection suggests the addition of docetaxel to 5-fluorouracil–cisplatin induction therapy may offer survival benefit in squamous cell cancer of the Head and Neck. *Palliative Chemother Anticancer Drugs*, **15**, 3331–340.

12 De Crevoisier, R., Bourhis, J., Domenge, C., *et al.* (1998). Full-dose reirradiation for unresectable head and neck carcinoma: experience at the Gustave-Roussy Institute in a series of 169 patients. *J Clin Oncol*, **16**, 3556–3562.

Chapter 4

Management of airway problems in advanced or recurrent disease

Nicholas Gibbins and Piyush Jani

Cancer is a word, not a sentence.

> John Diamond, C p. 17, Vermilion, London (1998)

We palliate what we cannot cure.

> Samuel Johnson, Dictionary of the English Language (1755)

Introduction

Head and neck cancer contributes 9500 new cases in the UK each year. The most common sites are the larynx, oral cavity, pharynx, thyroid, and salivary gland,[1] with the larynx being the most prevalent in the Western world. It represents 1% of all malignancies in men and is the sixth most common cancer in the Western world. In some areas of India and Malaysia, it is the most common cancer. It has a male to female ratio of 5:1. The incidence increases with age, but the peak presentation is in the seventh decade. The most common histopathology is squamous cell carcinoma (SCC) of the upper aerodigestive tract and is directly related to smoking. It is not directly related to alcohol intake, but alcohol intake is highly synergistic with smoking.[2]

At the time of presentation, many patients have advanced disease[3] and subsequently the treatment of patients with advanced or recurrent disease is a relatively common undertaking. The management of these patients presents the surgical team with unique problems, with a major difference from advanced cancers in other areas being that the area is visible to themselves, their family and friends, and the general population, and is difficult to shield.[4] Because of this, the psychological effect that head and neck cancer has on the patient can be magnified. The dying process tends to be slow and unpleasant, and it is essential for a multidisciplinary team approach to be taken when dealing with this.[5]

Multidisciplinary team

The multidisciplinary head and neck cancer team should include:

+ ENT surgeons
+ Speech and language therapists
+ Tracheostomy specialist nurses
+ Oncologists
+ GPs
+ District durses
+ Specialist palliative care team in hospital and/or community
+ Specialist psychological help, where needed.

Specific consideration should be given to the psychological distress, not only of the patient, but also of their family. This is especially important at the time of diagnosis and when treatment is to be changed to palliative, or when surgical or oncological treatment is withdrawn.

Treatment

The plan of management needs to be based on a number of considerations:

+ The patients' co-morbidities are always reviewed if any surgical treatment is being considered, not only from the view of the anaesthetic risk, but also the possible morbidity and post-operative recovery time related to the surgery that will be needed. Does the patient have the reserves to recover and benefit from the operation being considered?
+ The patients' lifespan with the disease must be assessed. This will be a major determinant as to which treatment modalities will be available for the patient.
+ The patients' expectation of their condition, their prognosis, and the time span of their disease are of paramount importance. This is a two-way information flow and must be kept up to date at each meeting (out-patients or multidisciplinary team).
+ Unrealistic expectations from either side (patient or doctor) leads to miscommunication and can result in fear of the unknown for the patient.
+ A careful consideration of what is possible, medically and surgically, for the patient against what is appropriate should be taken at each step of the care pathway.

What is possible ≠ always what is appropriate

Physiology

> While there are several chronic diseases more destructive to life than cancer, none is more feared
>
> Charles H Mayo, *Annals of Surgery* **83**: 357 (1926)

To consider the airway management in the patient with advanced or recurrent head and neck cancer, one must first understand some of the basic principles involved in airflow.

Laminar flow

The flow of air through the upper airways, like the flow of liquids through rigid narrow tubes, is normally laminar, or *streamlined* (see Fig. 4.1)

This resembles the flow of a river, where the air nearest the trachea walls moves more slowly than that in the centre of the airway. Laminar flow is maintained only up to a certain velocity. Beyond this, the flow becomes disrupted, or *turbulent*. In the same way that you can hear a stream, but cannot hear a river, one is unable to hear laminar flow, but one can hear turbulent flow, which manifests clinically in the upper airways as stridor and in arteries as bruits.

Stridor = presence of turbulent airflow

Another important physiological concept is that of the relationship between the flow in a long narrow tube (trachea in this case), the viscosity of the

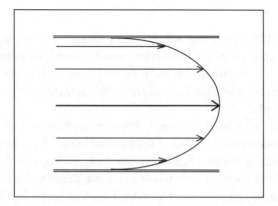

Fig. 4.1 Laminar flow.

substance passing through it (air), and the radius of the tube. This is represented mathematically by the *Poiseuille–Hagen* formula. The original formula is adjusted to give:

$$R = 8\eta L/\pi r^4$$

where R = resistance; η = viscosity; L = length of the tube;
and r = radius of the tube.

The important, and most variable, part of this equation is the radius of the tube, or trachea. The length of the tube, viscosity of the air, and the resistance remain reasonably stationary *in vivo*. The flow varies directly (and the resistance inversely) with the fourth power of the radius.

In other words, the flow through a tube is *doubled* with only a 19% increase in its radius. Conversely, if the radius of the tube is halved, the resistance, and therefore the effort of respiration, is increased by *16 times*. This goes some way to explaining why, when a patients' airway starts to become problematic, it can very rapidly turn into an emergency situation as a patient tires. This reinforces the need to treat airway problems early.

There is another aspect of this physiology that can be applied practically in clinical management. If the airway is narrowed and there is a delay before definitive treatment (for example, a tracheostomy for a laryngeal carcinoma), and the patient is starting to fatigue, one way to help the situation is to try and re-adjust the Poiseuille–Hagen equation. The length and radius of tube and the viscosity of the air (η, L, and r) cannot be changed, but the resistance of the airway is affected, not only by the *viscosity* of the substance flowing through it, but also by its *density*. The less dense the gas passing through the trachea, the less work is needed for it to pass along the tube.

Heliox

Heliox is a 21:79 O_2/He mix which has the same O_2 content as air, but the inert gas component makes the mixture much lighter. The atomic weight of helium is 4, that of nitrogen 14. N_2 in the atmosphere has an atomic mass of 28, seven times heavier than helium. *Heliox therefore reduces the effort of work needed to breathe.*

Heliox has been used in many different applications associated with airway compromise from asthma to stridor from burns.[6–8] All are based on the reduced density of Heliox. Higher concentrations of oxygen in the Heliox can also be obtained, the most common of which is a 40:60 O_2/He ratio.

The patient will get some relief from their work of respiration; however, the pathology causing the airway problem does not disappear. Heliox is, therefore, *a stop-gap procedure only* and in the emergency situation should not delay any surgical management needed.

Anatomy of airway obstruciton

Death is a debt we all must pay

Euripides—Alcestis 419

Almost any tissue in the head and neck can be the source of cancer, but those that can classically cause airway problems are those in the *larynx and the tongue base.*

Thyroid tumours can cause external compression or can directly spread into the trachea, neck metastases can similarly cause problems, and 'distant' tumours in the lung can invade the left recurrent laryngeal nerve as it loops under the arch of the aorta, causing a left vocal cord palsy (see Table 4.1). This

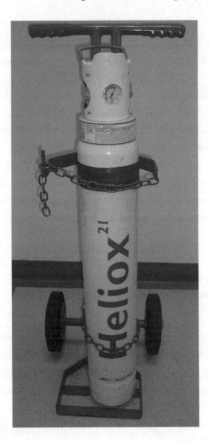

Fig. 4.2 Helioxcylinder.

Table 4.1 Head and neck cancers causing airway compromise[9]

Common	
	Larynx
	Tongue base
	Thyroid
	Neck metastases
	Lung tumours invading recurrent laryngeal nerve
Rare	
	Oesophageal
	Nasopharyngeal
	Oral
	Tracheal

will paralyse the cord in an adducted position, significantly reducing the cross surface area of the airway at the level of the glottis, leading to possible airway compromise.

More unusually, oesophageal tumours can spread directly into the trachea or cause posterior compression of the airway. By their anatomical location, nasopharyngeal tumours have to be large to cause airway problems but, if they do, the patient commonly has stertor (see below for definitions) as a presenting feature.

Oral carcinomas can cause airway compromise if there is a large intraoral component, such as a tonsillar carcinoma. Primary tumours arising from the trachea itself will cause stridor early, but are rare. Airway compromise caused by dental and facial/maxillary tumours is extremely rare.

Management

> Men fear Death, as children fear to go into the dark; and as that natural fear in children is increased with tales, so is the other.
>
> Sir Francis Bacon, Essays

The area of management which often provides the most difficult but the most important decision before undertaking surgery is that of patient selection.[10]

Conservative and medical treatment in advanced cancer of the head and neck will be primarily aimed at symptomatic relief, the most important of which is pain and the anticipation of it.[11]

Selection for palliative surgery will demand consideration of other physical and psychological factors:

1 The natural history of the disease in question must be known and appreciated. This will allow appropriate estimation of life expectancy and course of the disease.

2 Closely allied to this is the patients' psychological state and their wishes. The expectations and personality of both the patient and the family will also guide treatment and influence the post-decision or treatment state of mind.

3 The patients' physical status and concurrent co-morbidities will impinge on any decision to operate, whether the condition is elective or emergent.

4 Knowledge of all the treatments available with their associated morbidities and recovery expectations is essential.

5 Societal factors including culture, ethics, and legality.[12]

The acute airway

Pre-terminal event

The management of the acute airway in advanced or recurrent disease is different from that of the 'ordinary' patient only when death is close and it has been decided by all appropriate parties not to intervene with resuscitative measures.

It should be emphasized that the development of an acutely compromised airway as a patient is approaching death should be prevented. It is imperative to predict these situations and intervene proactively before this scenario arises, and discuss possible management strategies with the consultant on the specialist palliative care team.

At the end of life, pain relief and sedation should be kept very close at hand at all times, usually just outside the patient's individual room near the nurses station. They should have intravenous access kept patent with regular flushes. If the airway becomes blocked, make sure someone is with the patient at all times. Making contact urgently with a senior member of the specialist palliative care team is recommended to discuss management of any respiratory distress or

End-of-life medication

2.5–10 mg midazolam s.c. bolus/infused

2.5–10 mg morphine s.c. bolus/infused

0.5–2 mg lorazepam sublingually

Seek specialist palliative care advice.

Table 4.2 Treating the acute airway

Air of calm and reassurance
High-flow O_2 via a re-breather mask
Pulse oximeter to monitor oxygen saturation
Senior ENT and anaesthetic assistance needed
Heliox
4 ml of 1:1000 EPINEPHRINE with 4 ml of H_2O
β-Agonists, e.g. 5 mg of salbutamol
5–10 ml of normal saline

anxiety and the support of relatives. Pharmacological treatment could include subcutaneous administration of benzodiazepines (e.g. midazolam) and opioids (e.g. morphine). Lorazepam 0.5–2 mg sublingually is an alternative. Occasionally. i.v. drug administration may be needed but specialist advice should always be sought so that emergency treatment can be avoided. If necessary, small doses of i.v. midazolam (1 mg slowly and titrate as necessary) or (SL) lorazepam (500 micrograms) can be given initially, followed by prn doses of subcutaneous midazolam used PRN or by continuous in fusion. Morphine (or other opioid) may be necessary if there is respiratory distress.

Medical

At an earlier stage of the disease process, the acute airway must be treated with speed, but with an air of calm at all times. Reassurance is given. The patient is sat up and high flow oxygen administered via a Hudson re-breather mask. A pulse oximeter should be used and constant observations carried out. If the blood oxygen saturation remains below 95% then high flow Heliox should be administered (see Table 4.2).

If the patient is becoming fatigued, time is short and definitive measures (i.e. a form of surgical airway) must be taken.

A differentiation between respiratory distress caused by a *laryngeal* tumour and *pulmonary* dyspnoea or respiratory panic must be made,[13] and the differentiation between stridor and stertor will help aid this distinction and localize the area of obstruction.

Stridor and stertor

Stertor is the sound of obstruction at a level higher than the larynx (e.g. the oropharynx) and is inspiratory. This is usually due to large tongue base tumours and can be simulated by pinching your nose and trying to inspire

Table 4.3 Stertor and stridor

Stertor	Inspiratory
	Oropharynx
	Tongue base tumours
Stridor	Inspiratory—obstruction at the glottis
	Biphasic—obstruction in the upper airway (usually extrathoracic)
	Expiratory—obstruction in the lower airways (intrathoracic)

through the mouth with your tongue on the roof of your mouth or relaxed backwards in your throat.

Stridor is caused by obstruction at the larynx or below. It can be divided into inspiratory, biphasic, or expiratory (see Table 4.3).

Inspiratory stridor is caused by obstruction at the glottis (laryngeal cancers). When the chest expands to suck air into the lungs, negative pressure is created. This negative pressure pulls the laryngeal tumour inwards and closes off the airway. The larger the tumour, the more the blockage, the louder the stridor (until the patient gets tired). On expiration, positive pressure pushes the obstruction out and the airway is increased.

Biphasic stridor is caused by an obstruction of the trachea (this can be intra- or extratracheal). This lesion is equally obstructive on both inspiration and expiration. As the trachea is rigid, there can be no movement of the lesion and therefore no difference between the airflow on inspiration and expiration.

Expiratory stridor is caused by lesions lower in the intrathoracic respiratory tree. The most common version of this is the polyphonic expiratory wheeze of asthma. Air can get into the lungs with no obstruction from the upper airways as the negative intrathoracic pressure of inspiration opens the airways, but on expiration this process is reversed, the airways narrow and air is forced through smaller airways, producing the noise. Monophonic expiratory stridor, or wheeze, is the blocking of a single airway. When more than one size of airway is narrowed (e.g. asthma), a polyphonic wheeze is heard.

Flexible nasendoscopy is performed to assess the degree and the position of the obstruction. Intravenous antibiotics and steroids should be started to treat swelling and infection that may be superimposed on a necrotic area of tumour.

To minimize any negative pulmonary effect which might add to the patients respiratory distress, one can use nebulizers regularly. In these instances, senior, as well as anaesthetic, help should be sought early as the patient may require tracheotomy. The old adage 'the time you should do a tracheotomy is when you first think of it' remains as relevant now as ever before.

Surgical

Ideally, any surgical procedure should be done in a controlled environment, preferably theatre. This allows the operator good lighting, correct positioning and equipment, and trained assistance.

If an urgent definitive airway is needed, cricothyroidotomy can be performed.[14] However, there are instances when an emergency tracheotomy is preferred over a cricothyroidotomy. This is especially true when the patient is known to have a subglottic or large thyroid tumour.

Tracheotomy

There are three types of tracheotomy: *the percutaneous*, the *mini*, and the *surgical*, or *open*. The primary objective of all three types is to obtain a definitive airway. There are many reasons to perform a tracheotomy,[13] but the reason most relevant to this chapter is that of by-passing an upper airway obstruction (see Fig. 4.3).

The timing of performing the procedure affects the options open at that time.[15,16] There are three main categories to the timing: the *emergency*, *urgent*, and *elective*.

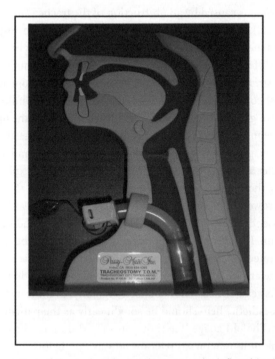

Fig. 4.3 Cross-section of the neck with a tracheotomy tube inflated *in situ*.

Tracheotomy is most easily performed if the patient is already intubated and under general anaesthetic as an *elective* procedure. This is the most common procedure and is primarily performed on patients who are having a tracheotomy for prolonged intubation (>7–10 days).

If maintenance of the airway is precarious and the patient is tiring, performing an *urgent* procedure under local anaesthetic is more appropriate.

When airway distress becomes an emergency and death is imminent, an *emergency* tracheotomy, or 'crash trache,' can be performed. This should only be done if intubation or cricothyroidotomy is impossible.[17]

Percutaneous tracheotomy

History First described by Sheldon in 1957,[18] and refined by Ciaglia *et al.* in 1985,[19] the use of this method of tracheotomy has increased in frequency over the last 10 years and is the subject of ongoing discussion and controversy (mainly between surgeons and intensive care doctors).[20]

Uses It is used most commonly in the intensive care environment, and the main advantage of many proposed by its proponents is that it can be performed at the bed-side with a lower risk of complications than open tracheotomy.[21] However, in a meta-analysis of tracheostomy techniques, percutaneous tracheotomy was shown to have a higher complication rate than open, or surgical, tracheotomy.[22]

Technique Whilst there are many different techniques, the underlying principles remain the same for all of them: entry to the trachea is obtained with a needle, a guide wire is introduced, and successive dilatations performed to produce a portal large enough to introduce a tracheotomy tube (see Fig. 4.4).

The advantages are that it is easier to perform, can be performed at the bed-side, and is more cost effective. However, the major argument against this

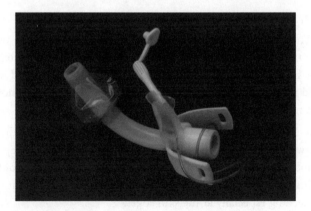

Fig. 4.4 Cuffed Portex tracheotomy tube.

method revolves around the fact that tracheal entry is obtained blind, without the pre-requisite of surgical procedures for exposure.

The potential complications are legion—the neck is surgical 'tiger country'—and can be catastrophic. Obese patients are particularly at risk. The risk of complications can, however, be significantly reduced by using concurrent bronchoscopic guidance to confirm entry into the trachea.[23]

As with any treatment course, patient selection is key. In experienced hands, the procedure is as safe as the open technique, but the operator must also be able to perform open tracheotomy in case the procedure needs converting.

Mini-tracheotomy

History Mini-tracheotomy, first developed by Matthews,[24] is usually used after operations (thoracotomy or laparotomy) for the treatment of sputum retention;[25] however, this is the most commonly used tube in the emergency scenario and can be used if needed in the short-term only.

Technique The main difference between a mini-tracheotomy and the other types is that the tracheotomy is performed not through the trachea but through the cricothyroid membrane. It is usually performed under local anaesthetic (remember sedation is contra-indicated in the hypoxic patient). An assistant is mandatory for this procedure. As with all types of tracheotomy, the neck should be extended by using a pillow or bag of fluid wrapped in a towel under the shoulders. Extending the neck exposes the trachea and helps keep it in the midline. The procedure is considered clean rather than aseptic.

The thyroid cartilage is felt and the cricoid just below it. A needle is passed through the cricothyroid membrane and air aspirated. A guidewire is passed followed by dilators. In elderly patients (especially men), the membrane may be calcified and may need to be incised. The mini-tracheotomy tube is passed over the wire into the trachea and tied into place.

Surgical tracheotomy

History There is evidence to suggest that tracheotomy has been used since before the time of Christ, but was used in a more widespread context for the first time in the diphtheria epidemic in France in 1825[26] and was even considered for George Washington.[27] Tracheotomy has steadily increased in use and is now a regular procedure.

Technique To perform a tracheotomy, as with all the types, the neck is extended with a support under the shoulders. The area is prepared and draped, and the midline structures marked (chin, cricoid, thyroid, sternal notch). Infiltration with a local anaesthetic/adrenaline mixture ensures reduced bleeding especially at the skin edges.

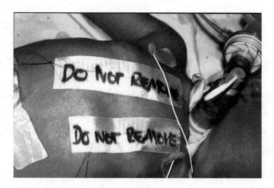

Fig. 4.5 Tracheotomy tube tied and taped in a neonate.

The tracheotomy tube is inserted through a horizontal incision half way between the sternal notch and the cricoid. The platysma is divided (absent in the midline), the anterior jugular veins divided, and the strap muscles separated, vertically, in the midline. The thyroid isthmus can be clamped, divided, and the stumps tied off. Once the balloon is inflated and haemostasis obtained, the tube is sutured in place to prevent accidental displacement (see Fig. 4.5).

When performing an emergency tracheotomy, it is important to note that the skin incision is *vertical*, rather than *horizontal*. This allows avoidance of the anterior jugular veins which run parallel to the trachea, and unnecessary blood which will obscure the operative view. Once the tracheotomy tube is *in situ*, haemostasis can be obtained, but this must not delay obtaining a definitive airway. Time is of the essence.

Vocal cord injection

Principles

Either recurrent laryngeal nerve, supplying the vocal cords, may be affected with parapharyngeal space tumours or with spreading cervical metastases. Alternatively a patient may present with a recurrent laryngeal nerve palsy if a pulmonary metastasis involves the left nerve as it loops under the arch of the aorta. Malignant disease accounts for 25% of all recurrent laryngeal nerve palsies, half of which are caused by carcinoma of the lung.[28]

The predominant symptoms that patients suffer from, associated with a vocal cord palsy, of dysphonia, aspiration, and stridor.

The vocal cords may be paralysed in the adducted or the abducted position and can give rise to different symptoms depending on which position the cords are paralysed in.

Unilateral abductor paralysis The single affected cord lies in the paramedian position (ADducted), and initial voice compromise may disappear as the ipsilateral cord compensates. Speech therapy may be the only treatment necessary.

If it does not improve, vocal cord injection may improve the symptoms.

If a patient presents with a left vocal cord palsy as the *only* sign, the diagnosis is commonly carcinoma of the lung, and the presence of recurrent laryngeal nerve involvement indicates that it is inoperable.

Unilateral adductor paralysis This is usually caused by damage to the vagus nerve, or both the recurrent laryngeal and superior laryngeal nerves. As the superior laryngeal nerve supplies the sensation to the larynx, and the recurrent laryngeal nerve the laryngeal sphincter, and these are both paralysed, aspiration may occur.

The palsied cord causes a quiet husky voice. Vocal cord injection combined with speech therapy for swallowing techniques can markedly improve the patient's symptoms and postpone the possible need for enteral feeding by nasogastric tube (NGT) or percutaneous endoscopic gastrostomy (PEG).

Posterior glottic incompetence can occur (a gap at the posterior edge of the vocal cords), but can be addressed using an arytenoid adduction procedure.[29] This procedure closes the glottis by rotating the arytenoid cartilage and suturing it in place. This rotates the arytenoids medially and closes the gap.

Bilateral abductor paralysis This lesion is usually idiopathic as a result of damage to both recurrent laryngeal nerves during total thyroidectomy; however, advanced thyroid cancers or bilateral neck metastases may rarely be the culprit.

The cords lie in the paramedian position (ADducted), and if the paralysis is acute at onset may be a life-threatening emergency and require tracheotomy. If paralysis is of more insidious onset, and the patient is immobile or sedentary, they may be able to compensate up to a point and there may be little stridor.

However, at some point, stridor and respiratory compromise will develop, usually associated with a respiratory infection. Many operations have been described to treat this problem, but if due to advanced or recurrent disease, *permanent tracheotomy* is the usual course of action.

Bilateral adductor paralysis Organic disease causing this is rare and is confined to neoplastic processes or other disease in the central nervous system. Most commonly, however, this is a presentation of psychiatric origin.

Medialization of vocal cord by injection

History

First described by Brünings in 1911,[30] injection of the lateralized vocal cord has been increasingly used over the last century. It has since been modified many times, and the number of substances used has been wide and varied,[31,32] but the current injection substance of choice is Bioplastic.

Uses

Vocal cord medialization by injection remains a standard procedure for laryngeal rehabilitation[33] and remains simple, has a low complication rate, and is highly efficient in *eliminating aspiration* and *improving voice quality and quality of life.*[34,35]

Technique

For the injection technique, the medialization material is injected either transorally or transcutaneously.[36] The injection substance is injected in the intrachordal space. This is between Reinke's space medially and the thyroid cartilage laterally. This is the space taken by the thyroarytenoid muscle which will have atrophied since paralysis.

Medialization thyroplasty

Medialization can also be obtained by inserting a Silastic or hydroxyapatite implant, or a Gore-Tex strip,[37] via an external approach through a fenestration in the thyroid cartilage. This procedure is usually reserved for patients with vocal cord palsies of aetiologies other than advanced or recurrent disease.

Laser debulking

History

Lasers were introduced to medicine from 1962 when one of the first reports was published concerning the interaction of laser light and living tissue.[38] The most common use of lasers in ENT is for recurrent respiratory papillomatosis,[39] but lasers have been used on laryngeal cancers since the 1970s.[40] In the 1980s, laser use expanded from excisional biopsies to include removal of tumours in a piecemeal fashion.[41,42]

Uses

Currently, transoral laser microresection is currently being used extensively for early tumours of the larynx and, in some anatomical types of tumour, it has virtually replaced some operations (in early glottic carcinomas, laser resection can replace hemilaryngectomy). In advanced or recurrent tumours there may be use for the laser as a more extensive method of treatment in the future, but at present *palliative relief of airway obstruction* remains the only use.

When a laryngeal tumour becomes large and inoperable, the airway may become compromised when the tumour grows to fill the glottis. If this becomes apparent, the *tumour can be debulked* using a laser. For the large laryngeal tumour which is threatening the airway, the carbon dioxide (CO_2) laser is used. The KTP (potassium-titanyl-phosphate) laser can also be used but is much rarer.

Technique

The laser is directed onto the larynx via a rigid non-fibreoptic laryngoscope. The operation is performed using the operating microscope. Possible fibreoptic technology is currently an ongoing research area. The advantages of precision, haemostasis, and reduced oedema allow an extremely neat operation via the intraoral approach.

The CO_2 laser produces light in the infrared range of the electromagnetic spectrum (wavelength $= 10.6\ \mu m$). This is invisible to the human eye and so a second helium–neon laser is used to make a red spot on the target tissue where the CO_2 laser will hit. This is used as the aiming mark for the CO_2 laser. The energy produced by the laser is strongly absorbed by soft tissues, independent of tissue colour, and the thermal effects on adjacent tissues is minimal. These attributes make it an extremely useful tool in Otolaryngology.

The KTP laser produces light at $0.532\ \mu m$ in the visible blue–green spectrum and is used for pigmented lesions as light from the laser is absorbed by haemoglobin and pigments, and causes focused protein coagulation.

Palliative laryngectomy

History

The first laryngectomy was, by all accounts, performed by Patrick Watson in Edinburgh at post-mortem.[43] The procedure was initially condemned, but once Billroth performed the first 'successful' laryngectomy in 1873 (the patient survived for a year, then died from a recurrence), the operation began to take root in the surgical psyche (Fig. 4.6).

Uses

Indications for laryngectomy have slowly decreased as an inverse relationship with the increase in surgical technologies for laryngeal organ preservation. The vast majority of the current indications are with *curative* aim; however, for some tumours, this is not possible but *surgical palliation* may be.[44]

With these patients, either anatomical (distant metastases) or histological (adenocarcinoma, spindle cell carcinoma, sarcomas, etc.) factors mean that cure is not possible with surgery, chemotherapy, or radiotherapy.

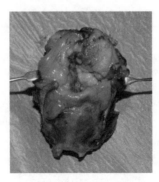

Fig. 4.6 A laryngectomy specimen.

Often, this group of patients have a combination of symptoms which cause particular problems. The symptoms that can cause significant problems and lead to a marked reduction in the quality of life include *dysphagia, airway obstruction ± aspiration* and *dysphonia*.

Dysphagia can be caused by a laryngeal tumour causing pressure effects posteriorly on the oesophagus, *airway obstruction* and *dysphonia* by tumour at the glottis disrupting the opening to the airway or the movements of the vocal cords.

In these cases, it is possible to alleviate these symptoms by performing a total laryngectomy as a palliative procedure.[45,46] Removal of the laryngeal tumour pushing on the oesophagus and glottis, and formation of an end tracheostomy solves the problem of the airway and dysphagia (see Fig. 4.7). In addition, once the patient has recovered from the operation, a Blom–Singer valve can be inserted to create a voice.

Summary

The treatment of the patient with advanced or recurrent head and neck cancer can be problematic and complicated; however, the management of the compromised airway in these situations can be broken down into two simple categories: the acute (needs attention as an emergency) and the chronic, or

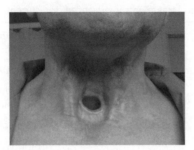

Fig. 4.7 End tracheostomy.

Table 4.4 Indications for tracheotomy[13]

Prolonged intubation	
Facilitation of ventilatory support	
Secretion management	
	Aspiration
	Bronchopulmonary secretions
Upper airway obstruction	
	Stridor
	Air hunger
	Retractions
	Obstructive sleep apnoea with desaturation
	Bilateral vocal cord palsy
Inability to intubate	
Adjunct to major head and neck surgery	

progressive, airway which needs urgent treatment. The management of the acute airway has very few differences from that of the non-malignant acute airway, but differences arise when dealing with the chronic airway.

Surgical management is often needed, but deciding if and when to operate can be the most challenging part of the patient's management. There is often no correct answer, but rather a series of options all with their own inherent risks and benefits. Weighing up the balance of risks of operation against the patient's health status and life expectancy is difficult, and one of many reasons why a multidisciplinary approach is used.

If intervention to the airway is needed and appropriate it should be carried out as soon as possible, but the key dilemma for the surgeon is the old adage 'it can take ten years learning to operate but a lifetime to learn when not to operate' (see Table 4.4).

Table 4.5 Uses of surgical treatments in advanced or recurrent head and neck cancer

Tracheotomy (in these cases)	To by-pass an upper airway obstruction (of any description)
Vocal cord injection and medialization thyroplasty	To medialize paralysed vocal cords
Laser debulking	Physically to reduce the size of an obstructing tumour
Laryngectomy	To alleviate problems which can arise with dysphagia, dysphonia, airway obstruction, and aspiration

These days the surgeon does not to make the decision alone but takes into account the patient's wishes, their prognosis, and the opinions of the multi-disciplinary team.

Case report 1

George M is a a 69 year-old man with a recently diagnosed glottic tumour for which he is about to start radiotherapy. He has quiet stridor.

Situation

A&E—4 a.m.

George has been unable to sleep and has real difficulty breathing when not bolt upright. He says his neck feels tight.

O/E:

accessory muscle breathing
loud inspiratory stridor
sats 93% on 100% O_2
resp rate 28/min
alert, but anxious.

George was treated with an *air of calm*.
Senior anaesthetic and ENT help was called for immediately.
I.v. access was obtained and he was given *steroids*.
Nebulized adrenaline and β_2-agonist were given.
A crash trache set and cricothyroidotomy equipment was kept within arms reach, just in case.

ENT assessment included *flexible nasendoscopy* which confirmed a large tumour at the glottis and a narrow slit for an airway.

The patient went *straight to theatre* for an *urgent tracheostomy* to by-pass the tumour. He had an uneventful recovery and was well enough to undergo radiotherapy the following week.

Case report 2

Rose, a 75-year-old woman, underwent a thyroidectomy and neck dissection for papillary carcinoma of the thyroid.

After the operation, she was unfortunately left with a unilateral (right) vocal cord palsy, but was otherwise well and went home.

Two months later, she re-presented to clinic with:

reluctance to eat
dysphagia
choking
hoarse, breathy voice
examination shows a paralysed right vocal cord in the abducted (lateral) position

Speech and language therapists assessed Rose but were unable to improve her symptoms with swallowing techniques.

Radiographic swallow and *videofluoroscopy* confirmed significant and constant *aspiration*. Rose underwent a *vocal cord medialization* with bioplastic injection.

Her dysphagia significantly improved and her voice partially resolved. Rose started to feel much better and her spirits improved when she started putting on weight.

Case report 3

Fred M, a 62-year-old man with inoperable laryngeal cancer was treated with palliative radiotherapy.

Later, he presented to clinic with *increasing dysphagia and breathing difficulties*.

A *tracheostomy* performed the same day as an urgent case relieved his breathing difficulties.

An NGT could not be passed past the tumour so a *PEG* was inserted. Fred recovered well and he went home with good support in the community.

However, Fred re-presented with the tumour encroaching on, and displacing, the tracheostomy.

After a long discussion with the patient and his family, the patient underwent *palliative laryngectomy* for symptom control.

End tracheostomy worked well and removal of tumour bulk improved dysphagia.

Once healed, a Blom–Singer (speech) valve was inserted and Fred got his *voice* back.

References

1 British Association of Otorhinolaryngologists, Head and Neck Surgeons (2000). *Effective head and neck cancer management second consensus document 2000*, p. 4. London, Royal College of Surgeons of England.

2 DeSanto, L,W. (1993). Cancer of the larynx. *Curr Opin Otolaryngol Head Neck Surg*, 1, 133–136.

3 Woolgar, J.A., Rogers, S.N., West, C.R., Errington, R.D., Brown, J.S., and Vaughan, E.D. (1999). Survival and patterns of recurrence in 200 oral cancer patients treated by radical surgery and neck dissection. *Eur J Cancer Oral Oncol*, 35, 257–265.

4 Pashley, N.R. (1980). Practical palliative care for the patient with terminal head and neck cancer. *J Otolaryngol*, 9, 405–411.

5 Rogers, S. (2004). Symptom palliation of diseases of the head and neck (including dentistry). In *Surgical Palliative Care*, Chapter 10, pp. 135–151. Edited by Dunn, G. P., and Johnson, A. G., Oxford University Press.

6 Rodeberg, D.A. (1995). Use of a helium–oxygen mixture in the treatment of postextubation stridor in pediatric patients with burns. *J Burn Care Rehabil*, 16, 476–480.

7 Austan, F. (1996). Heliox inhalation in status asthmaticus and respiratory academia: a brief report. *Heart Lung*, 25, 155–157.

8 Kitching, A.J., and Edge, C. (2003) Lasers and surgery. *BJA CEPD Reviews*, 3(5): 143–146.

9 Cawson, R.A., Binnie, W.H., Speight, P., Barrett, A.W., and Wright, J.M. (1998). *Lucas's pathology of tumours of the oral tissues*, 5th edn, London, Churchill Livingstone.

10 Goepfert, W. (2002). Advanced laryngeal cancer: current best management: 'the paradigm is shifting, but not much'. *Curr Opin Otolaryngol Head Neck Surg*, 10, 112–117.

11 Donnelly, S., Walsh, D. (1995). The symptoms of advanced cancer. *Semin Oncol*, **22**, 67–72.

12 Ng, A., and Easson, A.M. (2004). Selection and preparation of patients for surgical palliation. Ch 2 *Surgical Palliative Care*, pp. 16–32. Edited by Dunn, G.P., and Johnson, A.G., Oxford University Press.

13 Goldenberg, D., and Bhatti, N. (2005). Management of the impaired airway in the adult. *Otolaryngology, Head and Neck Surgery*, 4th edn., p. 2441–2453. Edited by Cummings, C.W., Flint, P.W., Harker, L.A., *et al*. Philadelphia, Pennsylvania, Elsevier Mosby.

14 Bourjeily, G., Habr, F., and Supinski, G. (2002). Review of tracheostomy usage: types and indications. Part I. *Clin Pulmon Med*, **9**, 267–272.

15 McWhorter, A.J. (2003). Tracheotomy: timing and techniques. *Curr Opin Otolaryngol Head Neck Surg*, **11**, 473–479.

16 van Huern, L.W.E. (2000). When and how should we do a tracheostomy. *Curr Opin Crit Care*, **6**, 267–270.

17 Goldenberg, D., Golz, A., Netzer, A., *et al*. (2002). Tracheotomy: changing indications and a review of 1,130 cases. *J Otolaryngol*, **31**, 211–215.

18 Sheldon, C.H., Pudenz, R.H., and Tichy, F.Y. (1957). Percutaneous tracheostomy. *J Am Med Assoc*, **165**, 2068–2070.

19 Ciaglia, P., Firsching, R., and Syniec, C. (1985). Elective percutaneous dilatational tracheostomy: a new simple bedside procedure: preliminary report. *Chest*, **87**, 715–719.

20 Hill, B.B, and Zweng, T.N. (1996). Percutaneous dilational tracheostomy: report of 356 cases. *J Trauma-Injury Infect Crit Care*, **41**, 238–244.

21 Massick, D.D., Yao, S., Powell, D.M., *et al*. (2001). Bedside tracheostomy in the intensive care unit: a prospective randomized trial comparing open surgical tracheostomy with endoscopically guided percutaneous dilatational tracheostomy. *Laryngoscope*, **111**, 494–500.

22 Dulguerov, P., Gysin, P., Lehmann, W., *et al*. (1999). Percutaneous or surgical tracheostomy: a meta-analysis. *Crit Care Med*, **27**, 1617–1625.

23 Barba, C.A., Angood, P.B., Kauder, D.R., *et al*. (1995). Bronchoscopic guidance makes percutaneous tracheostomy a safe, cost-effective, and easy-to-teach procedure. *Surgery*, **118**, 879–883.

24 Matthews, H.R., and Hopkinson, R.B. (1984). Treatment of sputum retention by mini-tracheotomy. *Br J Surg*, **71**, 147–150.

25 Bonde, P., McManus, K., McAnespie, M., and McGuigan, J. (2002). Lung surgery: identifying the subgroup at risk for sputum retention. *Eur J Cardiothorac Surg*, **22**, 18–22.

26 Borman, J.D.J. (1963). A history of tracheotomy: si spiritum ducit vivit. *Br J Anaesth*, **35**, 388–390.

27 Frost, E.A. (1976). Tracing the tracheostomy. *Ann Otol Rhinol Laryngol*, **85**, 618–624.

28 Stell, P.M., and Maran, A.G.D. (1978). *Head and neck surgery*, 2nd edn., pp. 194–204. London, William Heinmann Medical Books.

29 Isshiki, N., Tanabe, M., and Masaki, S. (1976). Arytenoid adduction for unilateral vocal cord paralysis. *Laryngoscope*, **14**, 555–558.

30 Brünings, W. (1911). Uber eine neue Behandlungsmethode der Rekurrenslahmung. *Verh Dtsch Laryngol Ges*, **18**, 93–151.

31 Montgomery, W.W. (1979). Laryngeal paralysis Teflon injection. *Ann Otol, Rhinol Laryngol,* **88**: 647–657.

32 Ustundag, E., Boyaci, Z., Keskin, G., *et al.* (2005). Soft tissue response of the larynx to silicone, gore-tex, and irradiated cartilage implants. *Laryngoscope,* **115**, 1009–1014.

33 Hartl, D.M., Travagli, J., Leboulleux, S., *et al.* (2005). Current concepts in the management of unilateral recurrent laryngeal nerve paralysis after thyroid surgery. *J Clin Endocrinol Metab,* **90**, 3084–3088.

34 Alves, C.B., Loughran, S., MacGregor, F.B., Dey, J., and Bowie, L.J. (2002). Bioplastique[TM] medialization therapy improves the quality of life in terminally ill patients with vocal cord palsy. *Clin Otolaryngol Allied Sci,* **27**, 387–391.

35 Flint, P.W., and Cummings, C.W. (2005). Medialization thyroplasty. In *Otolaryngology, Head and Neck Surgery,* 4th edn., pp. 2187–2198. Philadelphia, Pennsylvania, Elsevier Mosby.

36 Ward, P.H., Hanson, D.G., and Abemayor, E. (1985). Transcutaneous Telfon injection of the paralyzed vocal cord: a new technique. *Laryngoscope,* **95**: 644.

37 McCulloch, T.M., and Hoffman, H.T. (1998). Medialization laryngoplasty with expanded polytertrafluoroethylene: surgical technique and preliminary results. *Ann Otol Rhinol Laryngol,* **107**, 427–432.

38 Zaret M.M., Ripps, H., Siegel, I.M., *et al.* (1962). Biomedical experimentation with optical masers. *J Opt Soc Am,* **52**, 607.

39 Derkay, C.S. (1995). Task force on recurrent papillomas: a preliminary report. *Arch Otolarygol Head Neck Surg,* **121**, 1386.

40 Strong, M.S. (1975). Laser excision of carcinoma of the larynx. *Laryngoscope,* **85**, 1286–1289.

41 Steiner, W. (1984). Endoscopic therapy of early laryngeal cancer. Indications and results. In Wigand, M.E., Steiner, W., and Stell, P.M., eds. *Functional partial laryngectomy,* pp. 163–170. New York, Springer-Verlag.

42 Steiner, W. (1984). Transoral microsurgical CO_2-laser resection of laryngeal carcinoma. In Wigand, M.E., Steiner, W., and Stell, P.M., eds. *Functional partial laryngectomy,* pp. 121–125. New York, Springer-Verlag.

43 Stell, P.M. (1981). Total laryngectomy. *Clin Otolaryngol,* **6**, 351.

44 Sheppard, I.J., Watkinson, J.C., and Glaholm, J. (1998). Conservation surgery in head and neck cancer. *Clin Otolaryngol Allied Sci,* **23**, 385–387.

45 Bocca, E., Pignataro, O., and Oldini, C. (1983). Supraglottic laryngectomy: 30 years of experience. *Ann Otol Rhinol Laryngol,* **92**, 14.

46 Pradhan, S.A., D'Cruz, A.K., Pai, P.S., and Mohiyuddin, A. (2002). Near-total laryngectomy in advanced laryngeal and pyriform cancers. *Laryngoscope,* **112**, 375–380.

Chapter 5

Oral problems

Andrew Davies

Introduction

Patients with head and neck cancer can develop a range of different physical problems. Some of these problems are disease specific, whilst others are non-specific (i.e. present in all groups of patients with cancer). Moreover, patients with head and neck cancer may experience a number of contemporaneous physical problems.[1] Table 5.1 shows the prevalence of physical symptoms in a mixed cohort of patients with head and neck cancer referred to a pain clinic.[2]

The aetiology of these problems includes: (1) a direct effect of the cancer; (2) an indirect effect of the cancer (i.e. secondary to disability); (3) an effect of the cancer treatment; (4) an effect of a concomitant illness; or (5) a combination of factors.[3] Thus, physical problems may be present at any stage of the disease (at diagnosis, during treatment, during remission, or during progression) and may even be present following 'cure' of the disease. Table 5.2 shows the prevalence of

Table 5.1 Prevalence of physical symptoms in a cohort of patients with head and neck cancer referred to a pain clinic[2]

Symptom	Prevalence (n = 167)
Pain	100%
Insomnia	71%
Dysphagia	61%
Anorexia	45%
Constipation	31%
Dyspnoea	25%
Sweating	20%
Nausea	17%
Vomiting	14%
Pruritus	7%

physical symptoms in a surviving cohort of patients with carcinoma of the tongue (median follow-up of 5 years).[4]

Patients with head and neck cancer, like all patients with cancer, may report none, some, or all of their physical problems. The reasons why patients do not report problems are unclear. However, patients may not report a problem if they perceive the problem to be inevitable, if they perceive the problem to be untreatable, if they sense that health care professionals consider the problem to be unimportant, or if other problems/issues predominate.[5] Thus, it is essential that patients are specifically questioned about the presence of relevant physical problems.

The management of any physical problem involves: (1) assessment; (2) treatment of the underlying cause; (3) treatment of precipitating/aggravating

Table 5.2 Prevalence of physical symptoms in a surviving cohort of patients with carcinoma of the tongue[4]

Symptom	Prevalence (n = 29)
Xerostomia	100%
Dysphagia	76%
Fatigue	48%
Pain	43%
Insomnia	41%
Cough	36%
Drowsiness	34%
Taste disturbance	34%
Sexual dysfunction	28%
Numbness/tingling	27%
Dizziness	24%
Pruritus	21%
Anorexia	21%
Diarrhoea	10%
Sweating	10%
Weight loss	7%
Dyspnoea	7%
Constipation	7%
Nausea	7%
Vomiting	3%

factors; (4) symptomatic treatment; and (5) reassessment.[6] Assessment is required to achieve an accurate diagnosis, which in turn is required to determine the most appropriate form of treatment. In addition, reassessment is necessary to evaluate the response to the treatment (and any need to adjust or alter it). In many instances, radical treatment of the cancer offers the best opportunity for palliation of the symptoms.[3]

The focus of this chapter is on common oral problems encountered by patients with head and neck cancer, i.e. salivary gland dysfunction, taste disturbance, oral infections, osteoradionecrosis, and trismus. Readers are advised to consult one of the many comprehensive textbooks of supportive and/or palliative care for information about other (generic) problems encountered by patients with head and neck cancer.[7,8]

Salivary gland dysfunction

Definitions

Salivary gland dysfunction (SGD) is an umbrella term for the presence of either xerostomia ('the subjective sensation of dryness of the mouth') or salivary gland hypofunction ('any objectively demonstrable reduction in either whole and/or individual gland flow rates').[9]

Epidemiology

SGD is common in all patients with cancer, and very common in patients with head and neck cancer.[9]

Aetiology

There are a number of causes of SGD in patients with cancer.[9] The more important causes of SGD in patients with head and neck cancer are local tumour infiltration, local surgery, local radiotherapy, decreased oral intake, and drug treatment.

Radiotherapy

SGD is a predictable side effect of conventional radiotherapy to the head and neck region.[10] It develops soon after the initiation of treatment, progresses during treatment and for some time after it has been completed, and is essentially permanent. Various strategies have been adopted to try to ameliorate this problem, including the use of different radiotherapy techniques (e.g. intensity-modulated radiation therapy), the use of radioprotectors (e.g. amifostine), and the use of other agents (e.g. pilocarpine). The Cochrane Oral Health Group is currently evaluating the evidence for the use of various pharmacological agents to prevent radiation-induced SGD (Emma Tavender, personal communication).

Clinical features

SGD is associated with a variety of different oral problems.[9] Moreover, SGD may result in a more generalized deterioration in the patient's physical and psychological condition. The oral problems encountered in SGD reflect the various functions of saliva. The symptoms associated with SGD comprise xerostomia, oral discomfort, lip discomfort, taste disturbance, difficulty chewing, difficulty swallowing, and difficulty speaking. The signs/oral problems associated with SGD comprise dental caries, oral candidosis, and other oral infections. The psychosocial effects of SGD include shame, enhanced feelings of being a patient rather than a person, and a tendency to avoid social contact (particularly occasions involving speaking and/or eating).[11]

Management

The management of SGD involves: (1) treatment of the cause; (2) symptomatic treatment; (3) treatment of the complications; (4) general oral hygiene measures; and (5) specific oral hygiene measures (e.g. fluoride supplements, professional dental cleaning).[9,12] It should be noted that whilst it is usually not possible to treat the cause of the SGD, it is almost always possible to treat the symptoms of SGD.

The symptomatic treatment of SGD involves the use of saliva substitutes, or saliva stimulants.[9]

+ Saliva substitutes—water, artificial salivas (e.g. mucin-based, carboxymethylcellulose-based), other substances (e.g. milk, vegetable oil).

+ Saliva stimulants—chewing gum, organic acids (e.g. ascorbic acid, malic acid), parasympathomimetics (e.g. choline esters, cholinesterase inhibitors), acupuncture, other substances (e.g. sugar-free mints, nicotinamide).

The choice of symptomatic treatment will depend on a number of factors, including the aetiology of the xerostomia, the patient's general condition and prognosis, the presence or absence of teeth and, most importantly, the patient's preference.[9] There are good theoretical reasons for prescribing saliva stimulants rather than saliva substitutes. The saliva stimulants cause an increase in secretion of normal saliva, and so will ameliorate both xerostomia and the other complications of SGD. In contrast, the saliva substitutes will generally only ameliorate xerostomia. Furthermore, in the studies that have compared salivary stimulants with saliva substitutes, patients have generally preferred the salivary stimulants.[13] Nevertheless, some patients do not respond to saliva stimulants, e.g. some patients with radiation-induced SGD (see below).

Radiotherapy-induced SGD

The evidence for the use of parasympathomimetic drugs in the treatment of radiation-induced SGD has recently been evaluated in a Cochrane review (Andrew Davies, unpublished data). Only three studies fulfilled the entry criteria for the systematic review.[14–16] All of the studies involved the use of pilocarpine hydrochloride. The data suggest that pilocarpine hydrochloride was more effective than placebo, and at least as effective as artificial saliva. The response rate was 42–51%, and the time to response was up to 12 weeks. The side effect rates were high, and side effects were the main reason for withdrawal (5–15% patients taking the standard dose). The side effects were usually the result of generalized parasympathomimetic stimulation (e.g. sweating, headaches, urinary frequency, and vasodilatation). The response rate was not dose dependent, but the side effect rates were dose dependent, i.e. the higher the dose, the higher the incidence of side effects.

Taste disturbance

Epidemiology

Taste disturbance is very common in patients with head and neck cancer.[17]

Aetiology

The more important causes of taste disturbance in patients with head and neck cancer are local tumour infiltration, local surgery, local radiotherapy, SGD, and drug treatment.[17]

Almost all patients develop taste problems during head and neck radiotherapy.[18,19] It develops soon after the start of treatment (initial effect at ~1 week), progresses during the initial stages of treatment (maximum effect ~3–4 weeks), and varies in its duration (from a few weeks to permanence). For example, Maes et al. reported that 50% of patients had subjective taste disturbance 12 months post-radiotherapy.[19] The taste disturbance associated with radiotherapy is primarily the result of damage to the taste buds and/or SGD. However, other factors may be relevant in some patients (e.g. oral infection). It is likely that the contribution of these factors varies from one individual to another. For example, SGD is often an important factor in those individuals who have persisting problems.

Clinical features

Patients may complain of a number of different taste problems, including a reduction in taste sensation (hypogeusia), an absence of taste sensation (ageusia), or a distortion of normal taste sensation (dysgeusia).[17] Individuals with dysgeusia report a variety of different taste sensations, but invariably report that food tastes disagreeable. Patients may complain of a single taste problem (e.g. ageusia for all foods), or a combination of taste problems (e.g. hypogeusia for some foods, dysgeusia for other foods).

Taste disturbance may be associated with anorexia and weight loss. Furthermore, taste disturbance may lead to other disturbances of gastrointestinal function, i.e. reduced salivary gland secretion or reduced intestinal motility.[20]

Management

The management of taste disturbance involves: (1) treatment of the underlying cause; (2) dietary interventions; (3) zinc therapy; and/or (4) other interventions (e.g. complementary therapies).[19]

Dietary interventions

Dietary interventions include:[21]

- Consumption of foods that taste 'good'.
- Avoidance of foods that taste 'bad'.
- Use of additional flavouring (e.g. salt, sugar, and other flavours).
- Attention to the presentation, smell, consistency, and temperature of the food.

Ideally, a dietician should review all patients with taste disturbance.

Zinc therapy

Zinc has been used to treat taste problems in a number of different clinical settings. It has been found that zinc given during radiotherapy can limit the extent of objective taste disturbance, and also shorten the time to recovery of both subjective and objective taste disturbance.[22,23] Similarly, it has been found that zinc given post-radiotherapy can improve both subjective and objective taste disturbance.[18,24] However, Silverman et al. found that only 37% of patients given zinc supplements reported a subjective improvement in taste disturbance.[24] The aforementioned studies all used different regimens, and so it is difficult to recommend a particular regimen. (The author uses zinc sulfate monohydrate 125 mg three times a day for at least 1 month.) Zinc salts are generally well tolerated in this group of patients.

Oral infections

Epidemiology

Oral infections are extremely common in patients with head and neck cancer. In particular, patients are prone to dental caries (bacterial infection) and oral candidosis (fungal infection).[25,26] The other bacterial infections that may be encountered include the periodontal diseases and salivary gland infections.[25] The viral infections that may be encountered include the herpes simplex virus infections and varicella zoster virus infections.[27]

Aetiology

The underlying aetiology of these infections includes disruption of the oral mucosa, SGD, poor oral hygiene, poor diet (e.g. high sugar diet), and drug treatment (e.g. antibiotic treatment).[28]

Clinical features

The clinical features of these infections are similar to those seen in other groups of patients. However, patients with radiotherapy-related SGD often develop rapidly progressive dental caries, and dental caries in unusual locations (e.g. lower anterior teeth).[9] Dental caries may result in oral pain, and complications such as dental abscess, adjacent soft tissue infection, and adjacent bone infection (osteomyelitis).[25]

Patients with radiotherapy-related SGD often suffer from repeated episodes of oral candidosis. Oral candidosis may be asymptomatic, or associated with a number of oral symptoms (e.g. oral discomfort, taste disturbance). Moreover, oral candidosis may remain confined to the oral cavity, may spread locally to produce oesophageal candidosis, or may spread more widely to produce systemic candidosis.[26]

Management

The management of these infections is similar to that used in other groups of patients.[25,26] The immediate management of infection involves the use of appropriate antimicrobial therapy, which should be based on microbiological testing of appropriate samples (i.e. microbial identification and antimicrobial sensitivity testing).

The choice of antimicrobial therapy (where indicated) depends primarily on antimicrobial sensitivity testing, but is also affected by a variety of other factors, including the extent/severity of disease, the patient's preference about the available drug formulations, the patient's ability to use the available products, and the presence of relevant concomitant diseases and/or drug treatments.[25,26]

The subsequent management of infection involves the treatment of predisposing factors for the infection (e.g. SGD). Oral hygiene measures can be very effective in preventing the development of these infections.[12] However, the use of prophylactic antimicrobial therapy should be discouraged, since this practice promotes the development of antimicrobial resistance.[26]

In the case of dental caries, specific prophylactic measures include regular mechanical cleaning of teeth, chemical cleaning of teeth (e.g. chlorhexidine), fluoride supplements, and avoidance of high sugar foodstuffs.[12] Patients with radiation-induced SGD should be prescribed a high dose fluoride supplement. In the case of oral candidosis, specific prophylactic measures include mechanical cleaning of dentures and chemical cleaning of dentures (e.g. chlorhexidine).[26]

Osteoradionecrosis

Definition

Osteoradionecrosis (ORN) is defined as 'radiological evidence of bone necrosis within the radiation field, where tumour recurrence has been excluded'.[29] A similar phenomenon may occur in patients that have not received head and neck radiotherapy (so-called osteonecrosis).

Epidemiology

ORN is a relatively uncommon complication of modern head and neck radiotherapy.[29]

Aetiology

ORN is related to the late effects of radiotherapy on the bone (i.e. hypocellularity and hypovascularity).[29] As a result of these late effects, the bone has a limited capacity to cope with normal tissue turnover, and especially with tissue damage following trauma or dental extractions/other oral surgery. ORN usually occurs within 3 years of radiotherapy, although it can occur at any time following radiotherapy.[30] The mandible is much more susceptible to ORN than the maxilla.

ORN is affected by a number of different factors,[30] including:

- Radiation therapy-related factors—radiation dose, radiation fractionation.
- Disease-related factors—tumour size, tumour location.
- Patient-related factors—poor oral hygiene.

Clinical features

Store et al. have proposed the following classification of ORN:[31]

- Stage 0—exposed bone; no radiological signs.
- Stage 1—mucosa intact; radiological signs present.

- Stage 2—exposed bone; radiological signs present.
- Stage 3—exposed bone; radiological signs present; orocutaneous fistula; localized infection.

The clinical features are influenced by the stage of the process. Patients with early stage ORN may be relatively asymptomatic. However, patients with advanced stage ORN are usually very symptomatic (e.g. pain and discharge). It should be noted that the stage of the disease frequently changes, and may improve as well as deteriorate.[31]

The diagnosis/staging of ORN is based on a combination of clinical and radiological features.[30] Thus, patients with suspicious symptoms/signs should be sent for appropriate radiological investigations. Plain X-rays show decreased bone density, and may show fractures. Computed tomography (CT) scans show bone abnormalities such as focal lytic areas, cortical breaks, and loss of spongiosa trabeculation.

Management

The most important aspect of management is prevention.[29] ORN may be avoided if patients receive appropriate dental care prior to radiotherapy, maintain high standards of oral hygiene during (and following) radiotherapy, and avoid dental extractions or other oral surgery following radiotherapy. If dental extractions/other oral surgery are required following radiotherapy, then the use of hyperbaric oxygen can reduce the risk of developing ORN.[32]

In early cases, the management is conservative, and may involve removal of loose bone fragments, gentle sequestrectomy (i.e. removal of necrotic bone), irrigation, topical antiseptics, systemic antibiotics, and/or hyperbaric oxygen.[30] Other modalities that have been reported to be effective include pentoxifylline and vitamin E, ultrasound therapy, and electromagnetic stimulation. In advanced (symptomatic) cases, the management is surgical, and may involve either radical sequestrectomy or hemimandibulectomy with reconstruction.[29]

Trismus

Definition

Trismus is defined as an inability to open the mouth due to tonic contracture of the muscles of the jaw.[33] However, the term is used more generally to describe any restriction of opening of the mouth.

Epidemiology

Trismus is a relatively common side effect of the treatment of head and neck cancer (5–38% of patients).[34]

Aetiology

There are a number of potential causes of trismus in patients with head and neck cancer. However, the most common cause is a late complication of radiotherapy (3–15 months post-radiotherapy). The trismus is the result of fibrosis of the temporomandibular joint and/or of the muscles of mastication.[35] Not surprisingly, patients with certain anatomical tumours (e.g. nasopharyngeal, base of tongue) and patients treated with certain radiotherapy regimens (larger total dose, larger fraction size) are more prone to develop trismus.

Clinical features

The clinical features are very variable, and range from mild restriction of mouth opening with no associated problems, to almost complete restriction of mouth opening with major associated problems. The problems associated with trismus include difficulty eating (leading to malnutrition), difficulty swallowing (leading to aspiration), difficulty speaking, and problems maintaining oral hygiene (leading to oral infections). Not surprisingly, these physical problems may lead to psychosocial problems, particularly isolation and depression.

Management

The key to management is the early commencement of exercises to prevent the development of trismus (i.e. exercises that stretch the mouth/maintain movement of the jaw). It is recommended that these exercises be started at the end of radiotherapy, be performed regularly (10–15 times a day), and be maintained for a period of 1 year following radiotherapy.[35] It is important that patients receive ongoing encouragement to continue with this exercise regimen.

A variety of techniques have been used to treat established trismus, including exercise regimens (see above), mouth opening/stretching devices (e.g. stacks of tongue depressors, the Therabite Jaw Motion Rehabilitation System[TM]),[36] and various other interventions (e.g. pentoxifylline, microcurrent electrotherapy).[34] However, as with many other problems, prevention is better than cure.

Key points

* Patients with head and neck cancer may develop a range of physical problems, some of which are specific to head and neck cancer, and some of which can accompany cancer of any type. Oral problems are very common in patients with head and neck cancer.
* Many of these problems are chronic in nature, and are complications of the anticancer treatment.

◆ Many of these problems can be ameliorated by appropriate care before, during, and after the anticancer treatment.

◆ Most of these problems are amenable to treatment, although some of the treatments require specialist care.

◆ Physical problems can lead to psychosocial problems, particularly social isolation and depression.

References

1 Forbes, K. (1997). Palliative care in patients with cancer of the head and neck. *Clin Otolaryngol Allied Sci*, **22**, 117–122.

2 Grond, S., Zech, D., Lynch, J., Diefenbach, C., Schug, S.A., and Lehmann, K.A. (1993). Validation of World Health Organization guidelines for pain relief in head and neck cancer. A prospective study. *Ann Otol Rhinol Laryngol*, **102**, 342–8.

3 Roodenburg, J., and Davies, A. (2005). Head and neck cancer. In Davies, A., and Finlay, I., eds. *Oral care in advanced disease*, pp. 157–169. Oxford, Oxford University Press.

4 Harrison, L.B., Zelefsky, M.J., Pfister, D.G., *et al.* (1997). Detailed quality of life assessment in patients treated with primary radiotherapy for squamous cell cancer of the base of the tongue. *Head Neck*, **19**, 169–175.

5 Shorthose, K., and Davies, A.N. (2003). Symptom prevalence in palliative care. *Palliat Med*, **17**, 73–74.

6 Davies, A., and Finlay, I. (2005). *Oral care in advanced disease*. Oxford. Oxford University Press.

7 Berger, A.M., Portenoy, R.K., and Weissman, D.E. (2002). *Principles and practice of palliative care and supportive oncology*, 2nd edn. Philadelphia, Lippincott Williams & Wilkins.

8 Doyle, D., Hanks, G., Cherny, N.I., and Calman, K. (2004). *Oxford textbook of palliative medicine*, 3rd edn. Oxford, Oxford University Press.

9 Davies, A. (2005). Salivary gland dysfunction. In Davies, A., and Finlay, I, eds. *Oral care in advanced disease*, pp. 97–113. Oxford, Oxford University Press.

10 Guchelaar, H.J., Vermes, A., and Meerwaldt, J.H. (1997). Radiation-induced xerostomia: pathophysiology, clinical course and supportive treatment. *Support Care Cancer*, **5**, 281–288.

11 Rydholm, M., and Strang, P. (2002). Physical and psychosocial impact of xerostomia in palliative cancer care: a qualitative interview study. *Int J Palliat Nurs*, **8**, 318–323.

12 Sweeney, P. (2005). Oral hygiene. In Davies, A., and Finlay, I, eds. *Oral care in advanced disease*, pp. 21–35. Oxford, Oxford University Press.

13 Bjornstrom, M., Axell, T., and Birkhed, D. (1990). Comparison between saliva stimulants and saliva substitutes in patients with symptoms related to dry mouth. A multi-centre study. *Swed Dent J*, **14**, 153–161.

14 Johnson, J.T., Ferretti, G.A., Nethery, W.J., *et al.* (1993). Oral pilocarpine for post-irradiation xerostomia in patients with head and neck cancer. *N Engl J Med*, **329**, 390–395.

15 LeVeque, F.G., Montgomery, M., Potter, D., *et al.* (1993). A multicentre, randomized, double-blind, placebo-controlled, dose-titration study of oral pilocarpine for treatment of radiation-induced xerostomia in head and neck cancer patients. *J Clin Oncol*, 11, 1124–1131.

16 Davies, A.N., and Singer, J. (1994). A comparison of artificial saliva and pilocarpine in radiation-induced xerostomia. *J Laryngol Otol*, 108, 663–665.

17 Ripamonti, C., and Falfuro, F. (2005). Taste disturbance. In Davies, A., and Finlay, I, eds. *Oral care in advanced disease*, pp. 115–124. Oxford, Oxford University Press.

18 Mossman, K.L., and Henkin, R.I. (1978). Radiation-induced changes in taste acuity in cancer patients. *Int J Radiat Oncol Biol Phys*, 4, 663–670.

19 Maes, A., Huygh, I., Weltens, C., *et al.* (2002). De Gustibus: time scale of loss and recovery of tastes caused by radiotherapy. *Radiother Oncol*, 63, 195–201.

20 De Conno, F., Sbanotto A., Ripamonti, C., and Ventafridda, V. (2003). Mouth care. In Doyle, D., Hanks, G., Cherny, N., and Calman, K., eds. *Oxford textbook of palliative medicine*, 3rd edn., pp. 673–687. Oxford, Oxford University Press.

21 Twycross, R.G., and Lack, S.A. (1986). Taste changes. In Twycross, R.G., and Lack, S.A. eds. *Control of alimentary symptoms in far advanced cancer*, pp. 57–65. Edinburgh, Churchill Livingstone.

22 Silverman, J.E., Weber, C.W., Silverman, S., Jr, Coulthard, S.L., and Manning, M.R. (1983). Zinc supplementation and taste in head and neck cancer patients undergoing radiation therapy. *J Oral Med*, 38, 14–16.

23 Ripamonti, C., Zecca, E., Brunelli, C., *et al.* (1998). A randomized, controlled clinical trial to evaluate the effects of zinc sulfate on cancer patients with taste alterations caused by head and neck irradiation. *Cancer*, 82, 1938–1945.

24 Silverman, S., Jr and Thompson, J.S. (1984). Serum zinc and copper in oral/oropharyngeal carcinoma. A study of seventy-five patients. *Oral Surg Oral Med Oral Pathol*, 57, 34–36.

25 Bagg, J. (2005). Bacterial infections. In Davies, A., and Finlay, I, eds. *Oral care in advanced disease*, pp. 73–86. Oxford, Oxford University Press.

26 Finlay. I., and Davies, A. (2005). Fungal infections. In Davies, A., and Finlay, I, eds. *Oral care in advanced disease*, pp. 55–71. Oxford, Oxford University Press.

27 Bagg, J. (2005). Viral infections. In Davies, A., and Finlay, I, eds. *Oral care in advanced disease*, pp. 87–96. Oxford, Oxford University Press.

28 Brailsford., S., and Beighton, D. (2005). Oral infections—an introduction. In Davies, A., and Finlay, I, eds. *Oral care in advanced disease*, pp. 48–53. Oxford, Oxford University Press.

29 Chambers, M., Garden, A., Lemon, J., Kies, M., and Martin, J. (2005). In Davies, A., and Finlay, I, eds. *Oral care in advanced disease*, pp. 171–184. Oxford, Oxford University Press.

30 Jereczek-Fossa, B.A., and Orecchia, R. (2002). Radiotherapy-induced mandibular bone complications. *Cancer Treat Rev*, 28, 65–74.

31 Store, G., and Boysen, M. (2000). Mandibular osteoradionecrosis: clinical behaviour and diagnostic aspects. *Clin Otolaryngol*, 25, 378–84.

32 Feldmeier, J.J., and Hampson, N.B. (2002). A systematic review of the literature reporting the application of hyperbaric oxygen prevention and treatment of delayed radiation injuries: an evidence based approach. *Undersea Hyperb Med*, 29, 4–30.

33 Critchley, M. (1978). *Butterworths medical dictionary*, 2nd edn. London, Butterworths.

34 Dijkstra, P.U., Kalk, W.W., and Roodenburg, J.L. (2004). Trismus in head and neck oncology: a systematic review. *Oral Oncol*, **40**, 879–889.

35 Zlotolow, I.M., and Berger, A.M. (2002). Oral manifestations and complications of cancer therapy. In Berger, A.M., Portenoy, R.K., and Weissman, D.E., eds, *Principles and practice of palliative care and supportive oncology*, 2nd edn., pp. 282–298. Philadelphia, Lippincott Williams & Wilkins.

36 Buchbinder, D., Currivan, R.B., Kaplan, A.J., and Urken, M.L. (1993). Mobilization regimens for the prevention of jaw hypomobility in the radiated patient: a comparison of three techniques. *J Oral Maxillofac Surg*, **51**, 863–867.

Chapter 6

Improving swallowing and communication

Jane Machin*

Introduction

Head and neck cancer is particularly devastating because it can affect those two most basic and social of human functions, talking and feeding, and thus has far-reaching consequences for the individual's daily and social life.[1,2] Once the patient is receiving help from members of the palliative care team, it is likely that they will already know, and have been treated by, a specialist speech and language therapist (SLT). Both the effects of the treatments for head and neck cancer and the progress of the disease necessitate early input from the SLT, to help with both rehabilitation and maintaining function.[1]

This chapter describes the ways in which the SLT can continue to help as part of the multidisciplinary team, attempting to maximize the patient's remaining abilities, and compensate for other aspects of swallowing and speech function which may be impaired. The SLT will be working, like other team members, with a patient suffering increased discomfort or pain, and living with the knowledge that they are nearing the end of life. The chapter concentrates on the practical applications of the SLT's knowledge for swallowing and speech difficulties and does not give detailed information on the basic swallow mechanism, or the articulatory and phonatory system in humans. These topics are described in depth in standard texts (Logemann,[3] Groher,[4] Ashby,[5] and Ladefoged[6]). A separate section will deal with the potential specific needs of the laryngectomy patient who has undergone surgical voice restoration.

Multidisciplinary teams

Multidisciplinary teams offer many benefits to patients and clinicians alike. It is especially important to aspire to effective multidisciplinary teamwork for

* The author would like to acknowledge the advice offered by colleagues from several cancer centres, and the perspectives offered by patients and their families over the years. Both aspects have been of great assistance in preparing this chapter.

this patient group, as the expertise needed to deal with many of these patients' difficulties will require an overlap of knowledge and skills from different professionals.[7] Early referral is desirable and can sometimes be achieved through means of a dedicated AHP (Allied Health Professionals) clinic.

The SLT works closely with the dietitian, oral hygienist or dental specialist, and palliative care nurse specialist in particular[8]. The patient's wishes and needs and those of their family/carer should be respected as part of the team's work, and this can include discussing difficult choices (as each person may have a different perspective for the decision making), notably with regard to eating and drinking.[9]

Different team members will be involved to different extents at different stages of the disease trajectory. Much of the clinical consultation time of the SLT who works with head and neck cancer patients is devoted to giving and explaining information, discussing possible therapies, and listening to patient's preferences. There are some subtle differences in goal setting for palliative care patients, in contrast to those undergoing standard rehabilitation[8]. An awareness of the range of options for different eventualities may better prepare patients for any decline in function. Patients may find it helpful to focus on a practical skill, such as swallowing or articulatory exercises, to counter feelings of loss of control and increased uncertainty in their daily life. Advice, information, and supportive care can lead to better understanding of the anticipated disease course and the difficulties the disease and its treatment may cause. This helps if the patient needs to weigh up the relative risks and benefits of interventions the SLT might offer, especially regarding swallowing.

Swallowing

This is the aspect of care where multidisciplinary team working is so essential—many patients will have experienced a degree of dysphagia since diagnosis, if not as a presenting symptom, and as their disease progresses and the effects of various treatments also affect function, the combined efforts of SLT, dietitian, oral hygienist, and specialist nursing staff contribute to alleviate the problems. Other team members whose expertise on this subject may be required are the ENT surgeon, radiologist, and the restorative dentist or prosthodontist (where there are particular difficulties with dentition).

What type of problems might be expected?

It is accepted that the normal swallow can be divided into three overlapping phases, the oral phase, the pharyngeal phase, and the oesophageal phase.[4] Only the oral phase is under voluntary control. Head and neck cancer patients will frequently experience problems relating to the oral phase, such as difficulties with lip seal, tongue movements to control and manipulate the bolus, sensation, dental problems, difficulties chewing, and maybe difficulties with jaw opening. Some or all of these may lead to loss of control of the bolus and difficulty in transporting it through the oral cavity to the pharynx, also leaving the patient susceptible to aspiration of food and drink. Aside from the mechanical problems, patients can experience taste alterations and dryness of the mouth.

The pharyngeal phase may also be adversely affected owing to tumour progression, as well as surgery, radiotherapy, and chemotherapy, with resulting reduction in sensation and diminished muscular control and coordination, so again directing and transporting the bolus may be difficult.

Both oral and pharyngeal stage problems can place patients at risk of aspiration of food and drink, and ultimately of developing unwanted chest infections. Reduction in the efficiency of swallowing could well affect nutritional status. It is important to stress how closely the identified stages of the swallow are interdependent, so problems tend to be inter-related and rarely occur in isolation.

How can the SLT help?

The SLT will assess the patient's current swallowing status and needs by clinical bedside observation, but also use FEES (fibreoptic endoscopic evaluation of swallowing),[10] and/or videofluoroscopy (modified barium swallow) if insufficient information can be gained from the bed-side assessment.

Frequent monitoring and reassessment may be indicated as a patient's abilities and status fluctuate. Tiredness may affect swallowing capability: it is frequently a side effect of treatment and of the disease itself, and is a contributory factor to fluctuations in ability to swallow or may exacerbate difficulties. The patient's emotional status, pain control, and any nausea or constipation can also reduce the desire to eat.

The SLT will make recommendations on how to help minimize deficits or compensate for problems. Usually there are three main ways to do this:

• manipulate the progress of the bolus itself in terms of consistency and viscosity

• alter head and neck posture to slow or direct the passage of the bolus

• use specific therapy techniques which will be described later.

How does the SLT work with other members of the team?

The SLT assesses the safety and effectiveness of the swallow and level of risk of aspiration. It can be difficult to identify silent aspiration, and the implications of this need to be taken into account. The SLT shows the patient ways to modify their diet and use compensations and techniques to swallow more safely.

The dietitian makes a full nutritional assessment to ensure sufficient calorie intake, as nutritional problems are common for many head and neck patients,[11,12] and will often combine oral/non-oral feeding. It can be very time-consuming and fatiguing to eat and drink with an impaired swallow, so the use of alternative and supplementary feeding methods as well as the oral route can relieve the pressure on the patient in these difficult circumstances. The SLT and dietitian work together to combine their advice, suggestions, and expertise.

The oral hygienist can offer much help and advice about promoting and maintaining good hygiene in the oral cavity. This is reviewed in detail elsewhere.[13-15] Dysphagia may be exacerbated by poor oral hygiene, such as coated tongue, build up of plaque on teeth, and sore lips. As an example, xerostomia severely reduces the ability to swallow and is commonly associated with head and neck chemo-irradiation, and any patient who has had radiotherapy treatment which includes the mouth will have a greatly diminished volume of saliva (secretion may be reduced by as much as 50%[16]). The saliva also changes in composition, which in turn affects the pH of the oral cavity and the way the mouth 'feels'. In addition, the patient may also have to contend with ulceration and mucositis, and sometimes taste changes, which are other possible consequences of treatment.

Assessment procedures

Clinical bed-side assessment

This is exactly what it says it is—a thorough observation of the patient at bed-side including trial swallows. Most SLT departments have a favoured proforma, developed to suit the needs of their caseload, and for head and neck cancer there will often be an extra section to record site and staging of tumour, structural alterations post-surgery, and the presence of any flap repair. Details of radiotherapy fields and treatment dose, and any chemotherapy need to be noted.

Within the assessment, background information is gathered regarding general medical history, current diagnosis and treatment, and nature of the reported dysphagia. Some patients report loss of appetite as result of their disease and treatment. It is helpful to establish where patient and carer's priorities lie and to have an idea of previous eating and drinking habits, in order to establish appropriate goals. This may include a desire to get back to the pub as soon as possible, and in this instance giving the patient safe techniques is often the limit of what can be achieved.

Lip seal, dentition, tongue movements (including sensation, range, strength, and tone), jaw opening, and soft palate are examined, laryngeal function is identified by means of voice quality, swallow/cough, and a picture is established of where the difficulties lie. Respiratory status and function, as related to the swallow, are also noted. The patient may have a temporary tracheostomy *in situ*.

The patient's ability to follow instructions is also important. If they are very easily tired, it may be necessary to carry out the assessment in shorter sections, at separate times.

Trial swallows are carried out, often beginning with 5 ml of coloured water (so it is readily identified in secretions), but maybe using thicker liquid, soft semi-solid, or soft solid, depending on individual need and what the patient is currently managing.

If there is space on the proforma to mark off subsequent examinations, for example on a rating scale, useful comparisons may be made regarding alterations in function.

FEES—fibreoptic endoscopic evaluation of swallowing safety

This is important because it can provide information regarding anatomical changes in the laryngopharynx and how these might influence swallowing capability. FEES allows the amount of oropharyngeal secretions pooling in or near the laryngeal vestibule to be visualized; this has been demonstrated to be a predictor of aspiration. A limitation is that there is a 'whiteout' during the actual swallow as the investigator follows it on the screen. This technique is extensively described in the original article by Langmore *et al.*[10]

Videofluoroscopy (modified barium swallow)

This is performed with the help of a specialist radiologist, as an elective procedure, and has the advantage of offering a dynamic picture of the swallow, and an overall view of the swallow function and its difficulties is established. In some cases, it is possible and desirable to show this to the patient. It is a 'modified' swallow in that very small amounts of contrast are given as the focus is on showing how the different phases of the swallow link in with one another and the timing of any penetration or aspiration into the airway. It is also possible to visualize structural and mucosal abnormalities. Sometimes it is useful to see if a particular compensatory strategy or therapy procedure is having the desired effect, so therapy can be better planned.

However, it may not be appropriate for all palliative care patients, especially if they fatigue very easily, and a clinical maxim is that it should only be undertaken if it is not possible to get the information in any other way, and only if the clinicians feel that the result may change management.

What are compensatory techniques and therapy procedures (manoeuvres)?

Modification of consistency/viscosity

After assessment, it may be felt that a patient deals better with a particular consistency, for example that if liquid is thicker (or artificially thickened) then the patient will be able to retain better oral control of the bolus. Often, patients have difficulty managing 'mixed' consistencies (something which requires chewing, but has a runny sauce) as these are more difficult to control at the oral stage. The fact that a patient is having difficulty swallowing medication can easily be overlooked, but should always be considered. It may be possible to have a syrup-like suspension, or to swallow a small tablet within a bolus of soft semi-solid material.

What are compensatory strategies?

One advantage of these is that they are essentially quick to grasp and may take immediate effect; however, the SLT would wish to monitor the patient carefully to ensure continued usefulness. Here are a few examples

- The patient finds it hard to transfer the bolus through the mouth—try tilting the head back to utilize the effect of gravity; resume normal head posture when ready to swallow.

- The patient demonstrates a delay in triggering the pharyngeal part of the swallow (on videofluoroscopy, the bolus would pass the ramus of the mandible, but the pharyngeal swallow would not be triggered)—try the chin down posture.[17]

- The patient is known to have reduced laryngeal closure, resulting in aspiration during swallow—try the chin down posture, as this will put the epiglottis in a more protective postion and narrow the laryngeal entrance. If there is known weakness of one side of the pharynx, it may also help to turn the head to the affected side. This will increase the extrinsic pressure on the larynx and promote better vocal fold closure.

- The patient is known to have oral/pharyngeal weakness on one side (this would show up as residue on one side, on videofluoroscopy)—it might help to tilt the head to the stronger side and thus direct the bolus to the stronger side.

Some of the above examples show how information gleaned from videofluorscopy and FEES may prove helpful.

Therapy procedures (also described as swallow manoeuvres in the literature)

This means exerting voluntary control over the oropharyngeal swallow and thus altering the swallow physiology. One advantage of these is their effectiveness in reducing/eliminating aspiration. A disadvantage is that they may be unsuitable for a patient who fatigues quickly or finds it hard to follow instructions; they require sustained levels of concentration and muscular effort.

Here are two examples:

- Supraglottic swallow—this aims to prolong vocal fold closure and therefore initiates this closure before the actual swallow, minimizing the risk of aspiration during the swallow. The cough out, post-swallow, aims to clear any residue sitting above the airway.

- Effortful swallow—this attempts to increase pressure from the oral tongue and base of the tongue during the swallow, leading to a more efficient swallow. It may need to be coupled with a second clearing swallow, to help reduce residue, in order to be fully effective.

Both of these techniques could be visualized on videofluoroscopy, and FEES could provide biofeedback on the teaching of these strategies[18] and demonstrate any pooling of residue after an effortful swallow.

Factors which may interfere with effectiveness

Many patients in this group may have oedema in the oral/pharyngeal area as a result of tumour recurrence or progression, or as a consequence of surgery and/or radiotherapy. Clinically it has been observed that this can have a protective effect on the airway, but frequent monitoring by the SLT is advisable, as the amount of oedema may alter and then place the patient at risk. Occasionally, patients with recurrent oral cancer in the tongue/floor of the mouth may develop a myocutaneous fistula when at the palliation stage. This will impact on their ability to create the vacuum intraorally needed for an effective swallow and have implications for infection.

The description of the above SLT interventions serves to demonstrate that implementing these strategies may cause fatigue or be impractical, rendering total oral feeding an unrealistic goal. The benefits of alternative feeding regimens, used in conjunction with oral intake, are obvious, be the method nasogastric, percutaneous endoscopic gastrostomy (PEG), or radiologically inserted gastrostomy (RIG); the specialist dietitian will be closely involved with the patient (Chapter 7) and can advise on the relative merits and suitability for an individual.[19]

Ultimately, the goals for the patient should focus on improving or at least maintaining their comfort and safety and if possible help them retain some independence. Regular support from the SLT and dietitian allows their progress and changing needs to be monitored and recommendations adjusted accordingly.

How can communication be improved (including articulatory speech and voice)?

This is a broad topic and a crucial one—not only do many head and neck patients with advanced/recurrent disease have to contend with difficulties eating and drinking, they may also find it hard to communicate verbally. Ensuring patients have the best communication possible is one of the reasons why early involvement by the team is helpful, as the SLT will have established a rapport with the patient and their family/carer, and have a notion of their communication status prior to tumour progression or recurrence. This section deals with non-laryngectomy patients; the specific needs of patients following laryngectomy are covered in a later section.

Relatively little is to be found in the literature about *how* to help; there are some studies which include speech measures as an outcome for types of treatment.[20–22] The lack of information in the literature may be because these patients form a disparate group in terms of assessing their articulation. Many variables can come into play: the size and extent of the tumour, the type(s) of treatment, the patient's motivation, and the patient's communication needs.[23] Also, since dysphagia puts patients at risk of aspiration, rightly or wrongly, this can become the focus and priority of SLT intervention.

Normal articulation

Normal articulation for speech is dependent on many precise and highly coordinated muscle movements, primarily of the tongue, but also of the other so-called 'active' articulators. Active articulators are those which move, i.e. the lips, mandible, tongue, soft palate, and pharynx, and they work in conjunction with 'passive' articulators, which cannot move, i.e. the teeth and hard palate. The larynx is important in helping differentiation of vowel sounds, as well as producing the sound source for the voice[5].

The amount of resonance is also importance and will be altered further by surgery, or if oedema is present.

Evidently, a patient who has a tumour of the oral cavity/tongue and related structures may well experience difficulties with articulation, and these may range from slight to severe. Influencing factors will include:

- Tumour site and size.

- Surgical variables—the necessary sacrifice of cranial nerve branches for tumour clearance; oedema; further to surgery; or the type of flap repair, if there has been reconstruction. The effects of dental clearance and the effects of scarring.

- Radiotherapy variables—there may be oedema, fibrosis, dryness of the mouth, and a degree of trismus.

- Chemo-radiation—there are some reports of function being adversely affected by combined chemotherapy and radiotherapy regimens.[24–26]

- Tiredness—if a patient feels very fatigued, their articulation will also suffer.

What is alternative and augmentative communication (AAC)?

It is also important to determine the patient's motivation and to assess whether it is practical to work on specific aspects of articulation, to improve clarity, or whether in fact it may be necessary to introduce the idea of alternative and augmentative communication (AAC). AAC could simply involve using a 'magic slate', such as a mini wipe-clean white board, or a pen and paper, for difficult words; equally, it could mean obtaining and learning how to use an electronic aid, such as the Lightwriter®. For some patients, agreeing to try AAC will be a difficult step to take, as it alters communication from a two-way process to a three-way process. This can have its own frustrations. There is an AAC centre, where specialist advice can be sought for the suitability of different communication methods and aids an individual needs, in each geographical area of the UK. The specialist SLT will have access to that information and help, and will need to bear in mind levels of literacy of the patient, and the possibility of home devices for telephone use, such as amplifiers for weak voice.

Articulatory speech

In spoken English, there are four main points of contact between the tongue and the other articulatory structures, for the production of clearly differenti-ated consonant sounds. To achieve clarity of articulation, we need flexibility of all parts of the tongue[5], and speed of movement, as the tongue is also needed for vowel sounds. The shape of the tongue alters, to change its height and position in the oral cavity, when we produce vowel sounds; these are further modified by the amount of lip-spreading/lip-rounding.

There will be other articulatory differences for different languages.

For the patient with advanced/recurrent disease in the oral cavity/tongue, there may be difficulties with physically making these points of contact for consonant production, and with sufficient speed and altering the shape of the tongue for vowels. Altered resonance may make speech difficult to understand for the listener.

What can the SLT do to help?

Assessment will take into account those sounds which are difficult or impossible to produce, and the SLT will suggest ways of compensating for these and, sometimes, substituting them completely. Many of the assessment items from the bed-side dysphagia examination will be relevant—speech is a secondary function of the biological organs concerned. Once the SLT has a clear picture of what is difficult and has had a discussion with the patient about what they would like to improve, it is usually possible to devise some individual exercises for gentle, regular practice. Essentially, these management strategies are based on exercises which might be used with someone suffering from dysarthria, as the effects of the cancer and its treatment will be similar.

A range of motion exercises such as those used in dysphagia therapy can also be utilized to improve lip/jaw and residual tongue movement. Articulation exercises might include practising the sound as part of minimal pairs (where only one sound differs from the target sound), in different positions in words (initial, medial, final), and in connected speech.

For everyday purposes, even normal speakers do not articulate each individual sound—once in connected speech, sounds change, influenced by their phonetic environment, and the listener also has other clues, such as context, body language, facial expression, and so on. As an example of this, few people would say 'bread and butter', rather, [bɹɛ bmbʌtə]

Often, it is possible to compensate for difficult sounds, for example it is quite acceptable to a listener if the speaker uses [f] for [θ] and [v] for [ð], so for a patient who has reasonable lip mobility and intact dentition this is a suitable compensaton when tongue-tip to dental closure is difficult. Another example would be the use of the schwa sound [ə] to glide between difficult consonant clusters, or onto difficult initial consonants.

Sometimes, it is necessary to substitute one sound for another completely, in which the patient needs to get used to doing this consistently for it to be effective. An example of this would be replacing difficult [t] and [d] sounds with the glottal stop [ʔ] (a gap within a word, in place of a consonant).

The family/carer can benefit from explanations and advice from the SLT, such as slowing their own speech rate, reducing background noise, and being honest, without displaying frustration, if they have not understood. Also raising their own awareness of the importance of non-verbal communication, such as facial expression and gesture, is important.

The above examples give a brief insight into what is possible. In this patient group, therapy is being undertaken against the background of not expecting to improve in terms of disease status, but where the person may indicate their wish to do something practical and positive to improve their communication. Many patients work out their own compensations and manage very well; others ask for help and guidance and are keen to practise, within their capabilities and levels of tiredness. As with eating and drinking, they may wish to try to maintain oral communication, but, equally, they may accept the value of AAC to assist them. Other patients will opt for AAC methods at the outset. The SLT has the knowledge and skills to support them and advise them in their choice, so with the right motivation, they can alleviate their difficulties.

Surgical voice restoration (for laryngectomy) patients

Background

Surgical voice restoration (SVR) for laryngectomy patients as described by Eric Blom and Mark Singer has now been available since the early 1980s.[27] It is regarded as the best practice for possible communication options for the laryngectomy patient,[27] and the beauty of it is that it does not preclude the use of other communication methods, such as oesophageal speech and the electronic larynx. Its major advantage and outstanding characteristic is that it allows patients to speak fluently, using air from the lungs, and achieve an acceptable-sounding, functional voice. It is also reversible, should a patient decide not to continue using the prosthesis, or should it become necessary or advisable not to do so.

How does SVR work?

The essential principle of SVR is that it involves creating a puncture between the tracheal and oesophageal walls, ideally at the time of primary surgery.[28] This may, however, be carried out at a later date (when it is known as secondary puncture). As with any puncture wound, it will begin to heal if it is not kept patent. This role is fulfilled by the silicone voice prosthesis, which is essentially a one-way valve mechanism to allow lung air through into the reconstructed pharynx, whilst preventing aspiration of food and drink.

In order to use the prosthesis, the patient needs to occlude the stoma, thus directing air through the prosthesis and causing the muscles of the reconstructed pharynx to vibrate. This occlusion can be digital, or patients may use a 'hands-free' device, whereby the occlusion is achieved via the heat–moisture exchange filter (HME filter) they apply daily to the outside of their stoma.

The voice prosthesis is carefully sized and fitted for placement in the surgically created puncture. Healthy tissue will grip around the prosthesis, achieving a snug fit. The prosthesis is usually managed by the patient with specialist help from a suitably qualified SLT, specialist ENT doctor, and, sometimes, head and neck cancer nurse specialist. In straightforward cases, the patient can be expected to care for the prosthesis themselves with relatively little professional intervention, changing it as necessary; the frequency of changing is dependent on the type of prosthesis and other individual variables.

Surgical procedure

This is described in detail in a number of published papers, but for the purposes of this chapter there are three key factors during the laryngectomy operation which can contribute to functional voice and swallow, post-operatively

- The first is cricopharyngeal myotomy, whereby the muscles of the cricopharyngeus are divided, right down to the mucosal level, on one side. This then allows them to vibrate in response to air directed up through the pharyngo-oesophageal segment from the voice prosthesis.

- The second key factor is careful reconstruction of thyropharyngeus muscle, to help reinforce the reconstructed pharynx.

- The third is the reconstruction of suprahyoid muscles, which have been dissected off the hyoid bone, onto the repaired thyropharyngeus, effectively lifting and bringing forward the pharynx slightly during swallow. This may help to promote a more efficient post-laryngectomy swallow.

This is all described in detail in the Macmillan SVR Project course lectures.[29]

Patients with advanced/recurrent disease

Problems, however, can arise for the patient with advanced head and neck cancer, or recurrent disease. A combination of previous radiotherapy and/or disease may affect the properties of the tissue around the tracheo-oesophageal puncture (TEP) site, so that the puncture no longer retains the prosthesis firmly and there is obvious leakage of both food and drink around the prosthesis. This is potentially serious for two reasons. Quite apart from causing unpleasant coughing attacks, this escape of fluid into the lungs could lead to chest infection. Similarly, if the prosthesis becomes dislodged, it may fall into the airway, or the aspiration may reach greater proportions.

A comprehensive management procedure for patients experiencing leakage around the prosthesis when the tracheo-oesophageal party wall has become very thin (<8 mm) has been carefully described.[30] The same management principles would apply to our patient group:

- achieve a good fit initially
- avoid unnecessary changes
- attempt to shrink the puncture diameter by placing successively narrower gauge catheters
- maintain scrupulous cleaning procedures
- consider using a prosthesis with an extended phlange which might reduce peripheral leakage (this must be fitted by a suitably qualified SLT or specialist ENT surgeon)
- in very severe cases, consider using a cuffed laryngectomy tube; although it would not then normally be possible to use the prosthesis to help produce voice a cuffed laryngectomy tube with fenestrations will allow the continued use of the voice prosthesis.

A very specific procedure for the management of leakage around a prosthesis which is longer term in nature and has arisen prior to the recurrence of the disease has been described in the Macmillan Surgical Voice Restoration Programme lectures.[29]

The patient with advanced/recurrent disease may now be having difficulty using their prosthesis, but clinical experience suggests it would be preferable to try to keep it *in situ* and pay particular attention to cleaning and care. Psychologically, it might be detrimental to suggest removing the prosthesis if this has been their usual communication method. This needs to be discussed fully with the patient and their family/friends so they can choose their preferred option. At a time when things feel very out of control for the patient, they may like to keep some aspects as normal. It may be that their condition will fluctuate and that the prosthesis will work better at some times than at others. Clarity of speech using the prosthesis is affected, for example, by poor breathing (which would make airflow through the prosthesis weaker), or by excessive secretions pooling in the pharynx.

The usual removal procedure would be:

- discuss fully with the patient, their family/carer
- remove the prosthesis according to accepted best practice

- avoid giving food or drink to the patient for a couple of hours
- try some soft food after a couple of hours, then some sips of drink if no leakage is noted
- seek senior help if leakage is still observed after 5–6 h.

It may be that in patients with advanced/recurrent locoregional disease, a puncture would not heal quickly, or indeed if that tissue has been irradiated— in these situations the advice and help of a specialist ENT surgeon should be sought and a stitch might be needed. In extreme cases and depending on individual situations, the surgical raising of a sternomastoid muscle flap could be a solution.[27]

The latter is unlikely to be desirable or practical in a patient nearing the end of life. If this is so, then it might be possible to use a 'dummy' prosthesis, or remove the prosthesis and put a Foley catheter in its place, which could have the additional advantage of being useful for stoma-gastric feeding.

Patients who are no longer using a voice prosthesis/use other means of 'alaryngeal communication'

If the laryngectomy patient finds him or herself no longer able to use the voice valve, owing to the presence of disease in the reconstructed pharynx, the neck, around the puncture site, or in the stomal area, they will need to mouth words in an exaggerated fashion, sometimes known as 'overarticulation'. The SLT can offer help and guidance with this—if a patient so wishes. Where we would usually approximate the vocal folds (seen on fibreoptic endoscopy as a 'Y'-shaped true glottis) to produce a whisper, the laryngectomy will produce a voiceless whisper reliant on consonant differentiation to produce the different sounds, hence it tends to be both sibilant and staccato in nature. The vowels are harder to differentiate in the absence of an effective sound source.

Some patients might prefer to opt for the use of pen and paper, or an erasable 'slate', which is more laborious, but may be their preference.

Oesophageal voice production is dependent on a tonic vibratory pharyngo-oesophageal segment, as well as effective injection or inhalation of air fromthe mouth or nose. Thus, poor breathing at the advanced disease stage (which may translate into an inability to alter the pressures crucial to production of oesophageal voice) may affect the clarity of oesophageal voice, or indeed the ability to produce it at all. Copious secretions pooling in the pharynx will also reduce the ability of the tissue in the reconstructed pharyngo-oesophageal segment to vibrate effectively. As with the valve user, recurrent disease in the reconstructed pharynx or neck will also affect communication ability.

Users of the electronic larynx device may also find that the oedema which frequently accompanies advanced or recurrent disease will render optimal placement of the device and transmission of the sound difficult or impossible. For a patient who has neck recurrence, it might also prove difficult to find a good point for optimal placement, and in cases where there is a known risk of carotid blow out, or the patient has a fungating tumour, it may be too risky to continue attempting to use an electronic device

In these instances, the patient may require advice and support from the specialist SLT for overarticulation techniques and practice, as well as discussion regarding the use of pen and paper. It is also helpful to talk through these strategies with the family/carer, as patients can become very frustrated if family and friends 'second guess' what they are trying to say (however kindly this is meant).

Key points

- Early referral to the SLT is essential if the patient and family are to get the maximum impact of the range of treatments possible throughout the illness.

- Effective team working is essesntial as the patient's abilities can fluctuate markedly, and referral back when necessary is vital.

- There are many ways in which swallowing difficulties can be assessed and helped, and many of these are unknown to those working outside the area of SLT, so patients can miss out on potentially helpful treatments for this condition, if not referred.

- Patients who have had laryngectomies have specific needs, and early referral is crucial to effective management.

References

1 NICE (2004). *Improving outcomes in head and neck cancer: the manual.* p. 9 paragraph 2. London, National Institute for Health and Clinical Excellence.

2 Rogers, S.N., Fisher, S.E., and Woolgar, J.A. (1999). A review of quality of life assessment in oral cancer. *Int J Oral Maxillofac Surg,* 28, 99–117.

3 Logemann, J.A. (1988). *Evaluation and treatment of swallowing disorders.* Austin, Texas, Pro-Ed.

4 Groher, M.E. (1992). *Dysphagia–diagnosis and management.* Oxford, Butterworth-Heinemenn.

5 Ashby, P. (2005). *Speech sounds,* 2nd edn. Oxford, Routledge (Taylor and Francis Group).

6 Ladefoged, P. (2001). *Course in phonetics,* 4th edn. Fort Worth, Texas, Harcourt and Brace College Publishers.

7 NICE (2004). *Improving supportive and palliative care for adults with cancer: the manual,* pp, 134–137. London, National Institute for Health and Clinical Excellence.

8 Sullivan, P., and Guilford, A. (1999). *Swallowing intervention in oncology.* London, Singular Publishing Group.

9 Groher, M.E. (1990). Ethical dilemmas in providing nutrition. *Dysphagia,* 5, 102–109.

10 Langmore, S.E., Schatz, K., and Olsen, N. (1988). Fiberoptic endoscopic examination of swallowing safety: a new procedure. *Dysphagia*, 2, 216–219.

11 Forbes, K. (1997). Palliative care in patients with cancer of the head and neck. *Clin Otolaryngol Allied Sci*, 22, 117–122.

12 Shedd, P., and Shedd, C. (1980), Problems of terminally patients. *Head Neck Cancer Surg*, 2, 476–482.

13 Sweeney, P. (2005). Oral hygiene. In Davies, A., and Finlay, I, eds. *Oral care in advanced disease*, pp. 21–35. Oxford, Oxford University Press.

14 Eilers, J., Berger, A.M., and Petersen, M.S. (1988). Development, testing and application of an oral assessment guide. *Oncol Nurs Forum*, 15, 325–330.

15 While, R. (2000). Nurse assessment of oral health: a review of practice and education. *Br J Nurs*, 9, 260–266.

16 Davies, A. (2005). Salivary gland dysfunction. In Davies, A., and Finlay, I, eds. *Oral care in advanced disease*, pp. 97–113. Oxford, Oxford University Press.

17 Welch, M.V., Logemann, J.A., Rademaker, AW., and Kahrilas, P.J. (1993). Changes in pharyngeal dimensions effected by chin tuck. *Arch Phys Med Rehab*, 74, 178–181.

18 Denk, D.M., and Kaider, A. (1997). Videoendoscopic biofeedback: a simple method to improve the efficacy of swallowing rehabilitation of patients after head and neck surgery. *Oro Rhino Laryngol*, 59, 100–105.

19 Regnard, C. (1990). Managing dysphagia in advanced cancer–a flow diagram. *Palliative Med*, 4, 215–218.

20 Nicoetti, G., Soutar, D., Jackson, M., Wrench, A.A., Robertson, G., and Robertson, C. (2004). Objective assessment of speech after surgical treatment for oral cancer: experience from 196 selected cases. *Plast Reconstr Surg*, 113, 114–125.

21 Logemann, J.A., Pauloski, B., Rademaker, A., *et al.* (1993)., Speech and swallow function after tonsil/base of tongue resection with primary closure. *J Speech Hear Res*, 36, 918–926.

22 Imai, S., and Kenichi, M. (1992). Articulatory function after resection of the tongue and floor of mouth: palatometric and perceptual evaluation. *J Speech Hear Res*, 35, 68–78.

23 Rogers, S.N., Lowe, D., and Humphris, G. (2000). Distinct patient groups in oral cancer? A prospective study of perceived health status following primary surgery. *Oral Oncol*, 36, 529–538.

24 Kotz, T., Costello, R., Yi, L., *et al.* (2004). Swallowing dysfunction after chemoradiation for advanced squamous cell carcinoma of the head and neck. *Head Neck*, 26, 365–372.

25 Nguyen, N.P., Moltz, C.C., Frank, C., *et al.* (2004). Dysphagia following chemoradiation for locally advanced head and neck cancer. *Ann Oncol*, 15, 383–388.

26 Nguyen, N.P., Sallah, S., and Karlsson, U. (2002). Combined chemotherapy and radiation therapy for head and neck malignancies. Quality of life issues, *Cancer*, 94, 1131–1141.

27 Blom, E.D., Singer, M.I., and Hamaker, R.C. (1998). Tracheo-oesophageal voice restoration following total laryngectomy. Chapter 1, and Chapter 7, pp. 52–53.

28 Singer, M.I., Hamaker, R.C., and Blom, E.D. (1989). Revision procedure for tracheo-oesophageal puncture. *Laryngoscope*, 99, 761–763.

29 Course notes from Laryngectomy: Rehabilitation and SVR post graduate course at SCANAR (School of Cancer Nursing and Rehabilitation), Royal Marsden Hospital, Fulham Road, London SW3 6JJ. Available on SCANAR Intranet, 2006 (latest update).

30 Macfarlane, K., Moorthy, R., Clarke, P.M. and Edels, Y., (submitted for publication, 2006) "Management of Peripheral Leak - The Charing Cross Approach." *Clinical Otolaryngology*.

Chapter 7

Nutritional support for the head and neck cancer patient

Clare Shaw

Introduction

Nutritional screening, assessment, and implementation of appropriate nutritional support are an essential aspect of the management of the head and neck cancer patient. It is likely that patients will experience some difficulties with eating and drinking from an early point in their disease. However, as the disease progresses, so the difficulties with eating and drinking usually also progress.

Studies indicate that the incidence of malnutrition in head and neck cancer patients is 72%.[1] Malnutrition and weight loss may arise due to a number of reasons, which include poor food intake, and increased energy expenditure due to the physiological effects of the tumour, or the metabolic demands of the treatment. Nevertheless, poor food intake is the most common cause for malnutrition and weight loss in this group of patients (see Box 7.1).

Poor nutrition can have a major impact on the ability to undertake activities of daily living, on the overall quality of life, and also on the tolerance to treatment.[2,3] Equally important is the role that eating and drinking plays in the social activity of the patient's life. Each patient will consider eating and drinking from a different perspective, with some patients placing more importance on their need to eat and drink than others.

Assessment

Screening

All patients should undergo regular screening of their nutritional status with the aim of identifying patients who require a more formal nutritional assessment. Many of the routine screening tools employed rely on the patient's weight, their 'usual' weight, and/or their body mass index.[4]

In palliative care patients, the emphasis may shift away from using body weight and concentrate more on the patient's symptoms and quality of life.

Box 7.1 **Causes of malnutrition in patients with head and neck cancer**

Poor dietary habits

Anorexia

Difficulty opening mouth (trismus)

Dry mouth (xerostomia)

Oral discomfort/pain

Taste disturbance (dysguesia, 'mouth blindness')

Difficulty chewing (dymasesia), e.g. poor dentition

Pain on chewing, e.g. poor dentition

Difficulty swallowing (dysphagia)

Pain on swallowing (odynophagia)

Fatigue

Depression

Concomitant disorders, e.g. alcoholism

Social factors, e.g. low income

Questions directed at subjective weight loss, ability to manage food and fluids orally, and symptoms relating to oral intake should help to identify those patients who require additional assessment and support.

Nutritional assessment

All head and neck cancer patients should have access to a specialist Registered Dietitian as part of the multidisciplinary head and neck cancer team.[5] Such nutritional support is of particular importance during the acute stages of treatment, but is also of importance during the other stages of the disease (including the latter stages of the disease). Appropriate access to a Registered Dietitian will not only help to manage nutritional problems, but may also help to reduce hospital admissions for the purpose of feeding.[6]

A full nutritional assessment should be undertaken by the Registered Dietitian, and should include the following:

* weight
* weight history—subjective recall can be used, if the patient prefers not to be weighed
* dietary intake, i.e. food intake, fluid intake
* consistency of food tolerated/not tolerated, e.g. solid, semi-solid, pureed, liquid
* other characteristics of food tolerated/not tolerated, e.g. dry, moist, hot, cold
* symptoms relating to ability to eat and drink, e.g. poor appetite (anorexia), difficulty swallowing (dysphagia), dry mouth (xerostomia), oral discomfort/ pain
* biochemistry may be used to assess hydration (if appropriate). Additional parameters such as albumin are likely to be below normal, due to the disease process and not due to malnutrition.

It is often appropriate for the assessment to be jointly undertaken with other members of the team (e.g. Speech and Language Therapist). The role of the Speech and Language Therapist is discussed in more detail in Chapter 6.

Nutritional support

Dietary advice for the head and neck cancer patient should be based on a nutritional assessment, and also on the aims of supportive and palliative care. During the acute phase of treatment, the aim is generally to maintain or improve nutritional status, and to help the patient tolerate the relevant cancer treatment (e.g. radiotherapy). Whilst the same aims may exist for patients undergoing palliative care, the decisions about the nature of the intervention should be discussed in the context of the patient's wishes, their prognosis, and their ability to tolerate the more invasive nature of enteral tube feeding.

The approach to nutritional support should be a multidisciplinary one, with good medical symptom management, and appropriate advice/input from the Speech and Language Therapist. Nutritional advice should always be patient centred, and take into account factors such as food likes and dislikes, swallowing ability, home circumstances (e.g. ability to shop, ability to cook), and the ability to manage any additional feeding such as enteral tube feeding.

In addition, the focus needs to centre on anticipating problems with intake of food, fluids, and medicines, and to manage these proactively before the patient becomes too malnourished and frail. Once the patient is malnourished, then the risks of procedures such as insertion of an enteral feeding tube are likely to be higher than normal. (The risks of such procedures are already higher in head and neck cancer patients than in other groups of patients.[7]).

Oral feeding

In patients that are able to take their food orally, then advice may need to be given about the following problems.

Anorexia

Many patients experience a poor appetite, which may be related to an effect of the cancer, an effect of the cancer treatment, or to a variety of co-existent systemic and oral symptoms (e.g. nausea and vomiting, dryness of mouth). Advice about small frequent meals, appropriate food choice, and use of nourishing drinks may help to promote dietary intake in spite of the ongoing poor appetite. In addition, appetite stimulants such as progestogens and corticosteroids may be helpful, although the optimal dose, the time to start treatment, and the duration of treatment are still unknown for most appetite stimulants.[8] It is equally important that any reversible causes are adequately treated (e.g. antiemetics for nausea and vomiting).

Consistency and suitability of food

Food may need to be modified depending on the patient's ability to chew and swallow food. Thus, many patients will require their food to be made softer (e.g. pureed), or more moist (e.g. use of gravy/sauces), to allow them to be ingested. Pureed foods are often low in nutritional value unless high energy, high protein fluids are added during the blending process, e.g. milk, cheese sauce, or the proprietary energy and protein supplements. Certain foods may be particularly difficult to swallow, and so alternative foods should be suggested in their place.

Other patients will require fluids to be made thicker to prevent them from being aspirated. Proprietary thickening agents may be used to ensure that fluids are of the required consistency. Patients and their carers need instructions on their usage to ensure that the finished product is of the required consistency. Proprietary thickening agents may also be used to help to maintain the moisture component of pureed food.

Fortification of food to increase energy and/or protein content

Obtaining an adequate intake of energy and protein is particularly difficult if patients are eating small amounts of food, or are managing to eat only semi-solid foods or liquids. In such circumstances, advice should be given about fortifying the intake with ordinary foods and/or with nutritional supplements.

A number of foods can be used to increase the nutritional value of both savoury and sweet dishes. These may include the use of high energy and/or high protein foods such as full cream milk, cream, butter, milk powder, cheese, or oil. A number of proprietary food supplements are also available to fortify food. Patients and their carers should be given appropriate advice on the use of these different fortification measures (e.g. recipe leaflets).

Vitamin and mineral supplementation

If patients are managing an adequate dietary intake, then additional supplementation may not be required. However, many head and neck cancer patients will be following a limited diet, and will therefore require vitamin and mineral supplementation in the form of a once a day multivitamin tablet. (If patients are unable to swallow tablets, then an appropriate liquid supplement should be prescribed.) Alternatively, patients may take a nutritionally complete food supplement, which provides a combination of carbohydrate, fat, protein, vitamins, and minerals.

Use of nutritional supplements

Nutritionally complete supplements may be needed to help achieve an adequate nutritional intake. There are a number of supplements available on the market, but care must be taken that the correct supplement(s) is chosen for the patient in terms of its composition, taste, and texture. Table 7.1 has details on the different types of nutritional supplements available.

Some oral nutritional supplements have been produced specifically for patients with cancer cachexia. They contain n-3 fatty acids which, due to their anti-inflammatory properties, may help to reduce the metabolic element of cancer cachexia. A randomized trial in pancreatic patients produced interesting results, but failed to show that such supplemental drinks were any better at slowing down weight loss when compared with conventional high energy, high protein supplemental drinks.[9] Furthermore, poor compliance with the n-3 fatty acid supplemental drink was a significant factor in the aforementioned study. Currently, there are no published studies of the use of these supplemental drinks in patient with head and neck cancer.

Fluid intake

Many patients have difficulties in swallowing both liquids and solids (which may lead to problems with dehydration), whilst some patients have more difficulties in swallowing liquids than solids (which may lead to problems with aspiration). These features should be taken into account when

Table 7.1 Nutritional supplements

Type of supplement	Use/nutritional value of supplements
Nutritionally complete supplements, e.g. Ensure Plus, Entera, Fortisip	Designed to replace all food if sufficient volume is consumed. May be used as a supplement to food when total food intake is poor. Contains protein, fat, carbohydrate, fibre (some products), vitamins, and minerals in a liquid form. Often based on milk protein. Available in a variety of flavours both sweet and savoury. Usually provide 1–1.5 kcal/ml.
Energy and protein supplements, e.g. Build Up, Complan, Enlive Plus, Fortijuce	Used as a supplement to a poor food intake. Provide protein and energy but may not meet vitamin and mineral requirements. Often available as milk protein-based drinks, or fruit juice-flavoured drinks. Usually provide 1–2 kcal/ml.
Carbohydrate supplements, e.g. Caloreen, Maxijul, Polycal, Polycose	Available as a powder or liquid. Can be added to ordinary food and drinks. Provides energy, but no vitamins and minerals. Provides 3.75 kcal/g for powder and up to 2.25 kcal/ml for liquid.
Protein supplements, e.g. Maxipro, Protifar	Available as a powder. Can be added to ordinary food. Rarely used in isolation in cancer patients, who often require energy, vitamins, and minerals in addition to protein.
Fat supplements, e.g. Calogen	Liquid supplement providing additional energy from a fat emulsion (vegetable oil). Can be added to ordinary food and drink, or taken as a drink on its own. Provides energy, but no vitamins and minerals.

dietary advice is given, and also when considering the appropriateness of enteral tube feeding.

Symptom control

It is important that all symptoms are adequately assessed and treated. Specific dietary advice may be needed to be given for symptoms such as taste changes, dry mouth, or sore mouth (see Table 7.2). The medical management of these symptoms is discussed in more detail in Chapter 5.

Patients with dysphagia will require an assessment from the Speech and Language Therapist, who can advise on the consistency of food to be taken, and also on whether or not the patient is at risk of aspiration (see Chapter 6).

Table 7.2 Dietary management of eating difficulties

Symptom	Dietary management*
Anorexia (poor appetite)	Small portions of suitable food. Make use of 'best' (for eating) meal of the day. Encourage snacks between meals. Encourage foods which are enjoyed most. Encourage foods which are high in energy. Fortify food to increase energy intake, e.g. use of extra butter/cheese. Use alcohol as an appetite stimulant. Consider use of progestogens or corticosteroids.
Dysphagia (difficulty swallowing)	Small frequent meals of suitable consistency. Food may need to be pureed or liquidized. Fortify food to increase energy intake (see above). Thin liquids may need to be thickened with a commercial agent to overcome the problem of aspiration—needs an assessment from a Speech and Language Therapist. May require additional nutritional supplements if intake from food is inadequate.
Xerostomia (dryness of mouth)	Avoid dry foods. Modify consistency of food so that it is moist, e.g. use of gravies/sauces. Take food with small sips of water. Try tart foods, e.g. lemon, pineapple. Food may need to be pureed or liquidized to overcome the secondary problem of dysphagia. May require additional nutritional supplements if intake from food is inadequate. See Chapter 5 for further details of the management of xerostomia.
Taste disturbance	Encourage foods that taste 'good'. Avoid foods that taste 'bad'. Modify taste of food so that it is more palatable, e.g. use of salt/sugar. See Chapter 5 for further details of the management of taste disturbance.
Oral mucositis (treatment-related inflammation of oral mucosa)	Avoid coarse foods. Avoid hot foods. Avoid acidic, salty or highly spiced foods. Avoid dry foods. Modify consistency of food so that it is soft. Take food after taking analgesia. May require additional nutritional supplements if intake from food is inadequate. Such measures would be appropriate for other causes of inflammation of oral mucosa, and for inflammation of the pharynx and oesophagus.

* Dietary management should be combined with appropriate medical management.

Enteral tube feeding

Enteral tube feeding may be necessary for patients who are unable to take enough nutrition orally, for patients who are aspirating, or for patients who are at risk of aspirating. A proactive strategy should be adopted in order to try and avoid whenever possible their placement being done as an emergency procedure. It is essential that the use of enteral tube feeding is fully discussed with the patient and their carers.

The ability of the patient and/or their carers to manage enteral tube feeding should be considered by the multidisciplinary team. Some patients and carers may be taught to manage the feeding themselves, whilst other patients and carers may require substantial support to manage the feeding from district nurses when in the home setting. There are a number of different types of enteral feeding tubes, and their advantages and disadvantages should also be considered by the multidisciplinary team, and again fully discussed with the patient and their carers (see below).

Nasogastric or nasojejunal enteral tube

Nasogastric or nasojejunal feeding may be the route of choice for patients requiring relatively short-term feeding (i.e. for periods of <4 weeks). For example, it may be used in a patient with oral mucositis, where it is anticipated that the patient will return to oral feeding once the treatment has been completed and the mucositis has resolved. In addition, it may be used as an interim measure, whilst a more permanent tube placement is being arranged, or to improve the patient's nutritional status prior to placement of a more permanent tube. Fine bore tubes made from soft polyurethane or silicone are the tubes of choice, since they are more comfortable for the patient, and they are less likely to cause complications such as rhinitis, oesophageal irritation, and gastritis.

Placement of a nasogastric or nasojejunal tube may be difficult in some head and neck cancer patients who have altered anatomy as a result of their disease and/or the treatment for their disease (e.g. surgery). The correct position of the tube should be checked in accordance with local policy: a chest X-ray is considered the 'gold standard' method for checking the position of the tube. Care should be taken if the pH of the nasogastric tube aspirates is used as the method of checking the position of the tube, since a false-positive result may be obtained in patients who have been aspirating and who have gastric contents present in their lungs.[10,11]

All patients should be taught how to check the position of the nasogastric tube by either measuring the length of the visible tube or by testing the pH of the aspirate. Furthermore, all patients should be advised on what action to take in the event of their feeding tube becoming displaced or removed.

Gastrostomy tube

Gastrostomy tube placement may be considered in patients who are going to undergo extended periods of enteral tube feeding (i.e. for periods of >4 weeks). The two main methods for gastrostomy insertion are a percutaneous endoscopically placed gastrostomy (PEG) or a radiologically inserted gastrostomy (RIG). The tubes may vary in size from 9 to 22 Fr, and are retained within the stomach with a flange, balloon, or pigtail.

A PEG is the most common type of gastrostomy tube used for feeding, although this procedure may be difficult in patients with extensive disease, or a treatment-related stricture, which prevents the passage of an endoscope. Concerns have also been expressed about the risk of spread of disease during the insertion of a PEG (as a result of direct implantation of tumour). A number of case reports of this phenomenon have been presented in the literature.[12] When it is not possible to pass an endoscope, then an RIG should be inserted for the purposes of feeding.

Studies have suggested that head and neck cancer patients have a higher rate of gastrostomy tube complications than other groups of patients, with up to 42% of patients experiencing relevant complications in one reported series.[13] However, other series have suggested that the morbidity associated with a PEG insertion is approximately 10% in this group of patients: the most common complications are local site infection, granulation tissue around the site, migration of the tube, leakage, or bleeding.[14] Other complications which can occur include necrotizing fasciitis and intra-abdominal wall abscesses.

Once the gastrostomy tract has become established, then the gastrostomy tube may be replaced with a 'button' device: the button device lies flush to the abdomen, has an internal one-way valve, and requires the insertion of an extension set to allow feeding to take place. Insertion of the extension set requires a certain amount of manual dexterity on the part of the patient. Most buttons are held in place with an intra-gastric balloon that is filled with sterile water or saline. The intra-gastric balloon should be checked on a weekly basis, and this again requires a certain degree of manual dexterity on the part of the patient.

Jejunostomy tube

An enteral feeding tube may be inserted directly into the jejunum via a laparoscopic or open surgical procedure. This method of enteral tube feeding may be chosen for patients who have had previous gastric surgery, or who have experienced repeated aspiration after other types of enteral tube feeding. This type of feeding may be more time consuming for the patient since the feeding needs to be undertaken at a slower rate when it is given directly into the small intestine as opposed to the stomach (which has a larger capacity for the feed).

A range of ready prepared enteral feeds have been developed to meet the patient's nutritional requirements (if a sufficient volume is taken). They contain carbohydrate, fat, protein, vitamins, and minerals, and they usually provide 1–1.5 kcal/ml of energy; they are available in bottles or packs of 500, 1000, or 1500 ml. The patient's energy, protein, and fluid requirements should be calculated, and the feed planned to meet the nutritional requirements. Account should be taken of any oral intake, with the amount of feed being adjusted accordingly.

Various methods of feed administration may be used (see Table 7.3). The feeding regimen suggested for the patient should be appropriate to their lifestyle and home environment. For example, if the patient is still active,

Table 7.3 Methods of enteral tube feeding

Feeding regimen	Advantages	Disadvantages
Bolus feeding—volumes of feed administered via a syringe (e.g. 200–300 ml)	May reduce time connected to feed. Not necessary to learn how to operate a pump. Method can be used to give additional fluid.	Administration of feed or fluid may be time consuming. Increased risk of gastro-intestinal side effects if feed is administered too quickly.
Continuous feeding via a pump	Rate is controlled by pump. Reduction of gastro-intestinal complications associated with rapid administration of feed. Minimizes stress on cardiac,respiratory, and renal function.	Patient connected to feeding pump for majority of the day. May limit mobility if patient has to carry pump.
Intermittent feeding via a pump or gravity drip	Patient has periods of time free of feeding. Some patients may find gravity feeding easier than managing a pump. Some feed may be given overnight.	Increased risk of gastro-intestinal side effects if feed is administered too quickly.

then, wherever possible, feeding should not restrict their ability to carry on with normal activities. Additionally, if the patient is still able to take food and fluids safely by mouth, then enteral tube feeding may only be required at night as supplemental feeding. The method of administration should be discussed with the patient and their carers to ensure that it is realistic for them to undertake such a regimen on a daily basis.

The quantity of feed, and method of administration, should be reviewed regularly to ensure that it is being tolerated. Table 7.4 highlights some of the potential complications of enteral tube feeding, and also some of the potential solutions to these complications. If a patient's condition deteriorates, then the appropriateness of feed and fluid administration should be discussed with the patient and carers, and modified according to patient's wishes, and also the ongoing aims of feeding (see above). For example, a patient may decide they wish to reduce the amount of feed to enable them to have more time disconnected from the feeding pump.

Parenteral nutrition

Parenteral nutrition should only be used if there is no access to a functioning gastrointestinal tract. This is rarely the case in head and neck cancer patients.

Table 7.4 Potential complications of enteral tube feeding

Complication	Possible cause	Suggested management
Diarrhoea	Hyperosmolar feed	Reduce rate of feed. Reduce osmolarity of feed. Use fibre-containing feed. Antidiarrhoea medication. Exclude/treat other causes, e.g. infection.
Constipation	Inadequate dietary fibre Inadequate fluid intake	Use fibre-containing feed. Increase fluid intake. Laxatives or enema. Exclude/treat other causes, e.g. drugs.
Nausea	Rapid administration of feed Hyperosmolar feed	Reduce rate of feed. Reduce osmolarity of feed.
Aspiration	Reflux Displacement of nasogastric tube	Prop patient's head so there is a minimum of 45° of elevation between head and neck and thorax when feeding. 4 hourly aspiration to check gastric emptying. Post-pyloric feeding, e.g. nasoduodenal or jejunal feeding. Prokinetics, e.g. metoclopramide or erythromycin.

Key points

- The incidence of eating difficulties and malnutrition is high in head and neck cancer patients.

- All patients should be screened for malnutrition, and a full nutritional assessment given to those who are malnourished or at risk of malnutrition.

- Good symptom management is important to help patients maximize their dietary intake and improve their quality of life.

- A multidisciplinary approach is important to address fully all aspects of food intake and symptom control.

- Nutritional support in the form of oral supplementation or enteral tube feeding should be considered at an early stage. Late intervention may present more complications, particularly with enteral tube feeding.

References

1 Bozzetti, F. (2001). Nutrition support in patients with cancer. In Payne-James, J., Grimble, G., and Silk, D., ed. *Artificial nutrition support in clinical practice*, 2nd edn., pp. 639–680, London, Greenwich Medical Media Ltd.

2 Grobbelaar, E.J., Owen, S., Torrance, A.D., and Wilson, J.A. (2004). Nutritional challenges in head and neck cancer. *Clin Otolaryngol Allied Sci*, 29, 307–313.

3 Larsson, M., Hedelin, B., and Athlin, E. (2003). Lived experiences of eating problems for patients with head and neck cancer during radiotherapy. *J Clin Nurs*, 12, 562–570.

4 Ravasco, P., Monteiro-Grillo, I., Vidal, P.M., and Camilo, M.E. (2003). Nutritional deterioration in cancer: the role of disease and diet. *Clin Oncol (R Coll Radiol)*, 15, 443–450.

5 NICE (2004). *Improving outcomes for head and neck cancers. the manual*. London, National Institute for Health and Clinical Excellence.

6 Wood, K. (2005). Audit of nutritional guidelines for head and neck cancer patients undergoing radiotherapy. *J Hum Nutr Diet*, 18, 343–351.

7 Walton, G.M. (1999). Complications of percutaneous gastrostomy in patients with head and neck cancer—an analysis of 42 consecutive patients. *Ann R Coll Surg Engl*, 81, 272–276.

8 Yavuzsen, T., Davis, M.P., Walsh, D., LeGrand, S., and Lagman, R. (2005). Systematic review of the treatment of cancer-associated anorexia and weight loss. *J Clin Oncol*, 23, 8500–8511.

9 Fearon, K.C., Von Meyenfeldt, M.F., Moses, A.G., *et al.* (2003). Effect of a protein and energy dense N-3 fatty acid enriched oral supplement on loss of weight and lean tissue in cancer cachexia: a randomised double blind trial. *Gut*, 52, 1479–1486.

10 Dougherty, L., and Lister, S. (2004). *The Royal Marsden Hospital manual of clinical nursing procedures*, 6th edn. Oxford, Blackwell Publishing.

11 **National Patient Safety Agency** (2005). NPSA issues new safety advice to NHS on reducing the harm caused by misplaced nasogastric feeding tubes. Available from: www.npsa.nhs.uk

12 **Adelson, R.T., and Ducic, Y.** (2005). Metastatic head and neck carcinoma to a percutaneous endoscopic gastrostomy site. *Head Neck*, 27, 339–343.

13 **Ehrsson, Y.T., Langius-Eklof, A., Bark, T., and Laurell, G.** (2004). Percutaneous endoscopic gastrostomy (PEG)—a long-term follow-up study in head and neck cancer patients. *Clin Otolaryngol Allied Sci*, 29, 740–746.

14 **Baredes, S., Behin, D., and Deitch, E.** (2004). Percutaneous endoscopic gastrostomy tube feeding in patients with head and neck cancer. *Ear Nose Throat J*, 83, 417–419.

Chapter 8

Complex wounds in head and neck cancer

Diane Laverty

Introduction

Complex wounds in head and neck cancer are usually due to advanced disease. Patients undergo several forms of curative treatment which may leave their skin in a fragile and vulnerable state. In addition, tumours of the head and neck region may continue to grow despite several modes of treatment. Due to the limited tissue space, active tumours may protrude through the skin, causing numerous problems and symptoms.

The aim of this chapter is to explore the aetiology of and treatment options for these complex wounds. The symptoms that may arise and management of these will be discussed. Finally the impact that these wounds have on the patient's life will be reviewed.

Complex wounds

A cancerous wound that breaks through the surface of the skin is termed a *fungating wound*. They arise as a result of infiltration of the skin by malignant cells. These cells may arise from a primary skin tumour, an underlying malignant tumour, or through metastatic spread from a distant malignant tumour.[1,2]

They ulcerate through the skin and characteristically have a cauliflower appearance. As they continue to grow, they often invade adjacent structures or organs. Tumour infiltration of the skin involves the spread of malignant cells along pathways such as tissue planes, blood and lymph capillaries, and in the perineural spaces. The tumour can develop its own blood supply which may cause bleeding to occur locally. The blood supply may be outgrown as the tumour continues to grow, resulting in necrosis occurring.[3]

Incidence

There are no population-based registries that accurately document the incidence of fungating wounds;[4] however, a well documented study was conducted by Thomas.[5] He obtained a list of the radiotherapy centres in the UK from the Department of Health and approached the consultants working in these units. He received responses to his questionnaires from 31 out of 54 centres. His results indicated that the number of patients being treated with a fungating wound was 295 in 1 month and 2417 over a year. Head and neck tumours represented 24% of those patients, which is disproportionate to the incidence of all tumours. His conclusion was that 'these wounds occurred in sufficient numbers to represent a significant problem'.[5] Clearly these are quite old data and did not include in-patient, out-patient, day care, and

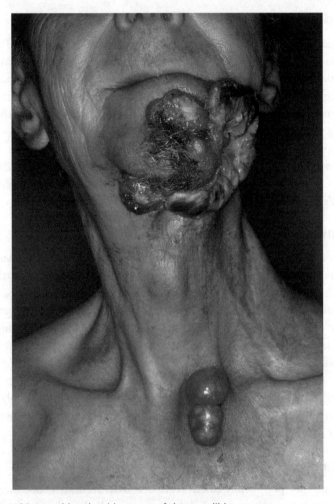

Fig. 8.1 A 66-year-old male with cancer of the mandible.

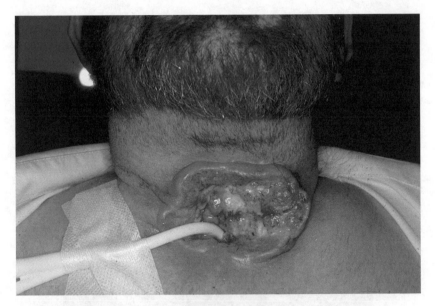

Fig. 8.2 A 58-year-old male with cancer of the trachea.

chemotherapy settings, but they allow us some insight into the incidence of fungating wounds.

A later study by Schwarz[6] demonstrated that fungating wounds occurred in up to 9% of all cancer patients.

There are no studies available that specifically focus on malignant wounds in head and neck cancer.

Aims of treatment

Unlike normal wounds, malignant fungating wounds rarely heal. The progression of their fungation may be impeded with the use of anticancer therapies, but the overall aim of wound management is:

♦ specific individualized symptom control

♦ promotion of comfort

♦ maintaining/improving quality of life.[7,8]

It must be explained to the patient that cure is no longer a possible option. The focus of care must be firmly directed towards the patient's needs and presenting symptoms. Psychological support for the patient is an important aspect of the nurse's role in caring for these patients.[8]

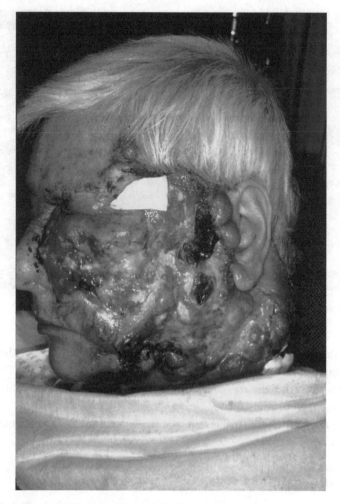

Fig. 8.3 A 61-year-old female with Merkel cell tumour.

Oncological treatment options

The use of oncological modes of treatment is focused on control of the wound and/or symptoms. The risks and possible benefits of all treatments should be weighed to ensure there is no deterioration in the patient's condition.

Chemotherapy

Single-agent or low dose chemotherapy may benefit by reducing some symptoms, e.g. exudates, but its suitability will depend on prior treatment the patient has received.[9]

Radiotherapy

Radiotherapy is the most useful palliative measure to control symptoms because it acts by destroying tumour cells and thus reduces the mass of the lesion.[9] Single-fraction or divided doses over 2–3 weeks may be used to reduce exudate, control bleeding, and alleviate pain. If fungation has not yet occurred, it may also delay this happening.[10]

It is important to note that any radiation therapy has the potential to cause skin reactions such as dry desquamation and erythema. These need to be treated according to local guidelines, and treatment should never cause further distress to the patient.

Surgery

This modality is rarely used in fungating wounds due to their friability and the local extension of the wound involving underlying structures. In certain circumstances, it may be possible to remove the lesion and use plastic surgery for repair, but usually the patient with head and neck cancer has already exhausted this option and further surgical resections would be inappropriate and unhelpful.

Symptomatic issues

Individualized symptom control of the malignant fungating lesion should be the main focus of care. Clinicians should possess the knowledge and skills to provide relief from symptoms and start the treatment for a complex wound. All teams should have a specialist or access to a specialist in this area.

Assessment

Assessment is the basis of good quality nursing care and the mainstay of evidence-based management.

Grocott[11] referred to the importance of assessment being patient focused. It should be guided by the patient who identifies the problems that are most troublesome to them. In conjunction with the professional's clinical assessment and concerns, this should form the basis of the initial and ongoing assessment.

Assessment of these wounds may take time. Once the health care professional possesses the appropriate knowledge of dressings, it is simple practice to match the symptomatic needs with the products available on the market. What often may take more skill and time are the psychological issues that the patient is confronted with. In the author's experience, a thorough psychological assessment may take up to 1 h.

In order to conduct a full and comprehensive assessment, it may be necessary to admit the patient for a short period of time. This allows the health care professional an opportunity to seek advice from a specialist practitioner, if necessary, and establish a relationship with the patient.

Symptoms will vary depending on the extent of the disease, size of the wound, and anatomical position. In addition, the patient's performance status and well-being can be important factors in their ability to deal with the wound.[10,11]

Symptoms rarely occur in isolation and, once they are resolved, more may occur. Management of these wounds is about constant reassessment and tailoring management to meet these changing needs.

Cleansing

Wound cleansing can be achieved with gentle irrigation to avoid further trauma, pain, or bleeding. Normal saline 0.9% at room temperature is the recommended solution,[12] and this should be performed with a syringe using gentle pressure.

It is also acceptable to encourage the patient, if possible, to shower the area gently during normal bathing,

Topical antiseptic solutions are not recommended as they may cause additional irritation or damage to the wound or surrounding skin.[13,14]

Exudate

Exudate production is due to the increased permeability to fibrinogen and plasma colloid of the tumour microvasculature.[9] Coupled with the fact that some tumours secrete vascular permeability factor (VPF), this may account for the large amount of exudate produced from some wounds.

Wound infection will also increase production and viscosity of exudate due to a prolonged inflammatory process.[12]

Excessive exudate can lead to peri-wound excoriation and leakage through dressings, which will adversely affect the patient's normal activity and quality of life.

It is important to choose a dressing that maintains a moist wound environment at the wound bed but is able to contain excessive amounts of exudate (see Table 8.1).

Alginates (e.g. Sorbsan, Kaltostat) and *hydrofibre* dressings (e.g. Aquacel) are useful in absorbing medium to high amounts of exudate. They are available in sheets and ribbon preparations and are on the Drug Tariff (i.e. prescribable on the NHS in the UK).

Table 8.1 Exudate reference table

Low exudate	Medium to high exudate
Alginate	Alginate
Foam	Hydrofibre
Non-adherent contact + absorbent pad	Foam
Stoma appliance	Stoma appliance
Non-alcohol skin barrier film	Wound manager appliance
	Non-alcohol skin barrier film

Foams (e.g. Allevyn, Tielle Plus) can be used as primary or secondary dressings in combination with other dressings. The foam needs adequately to cover the wound, allowing for a margin, and be comfortable when it is secured appropriately.[10] It is important to resist the temptation to use several pads for absorbency. These add to the bulky appearance and adversely affect the cosmetic effect for these patients. Grocott[15] suggests the use of a *non-adherent contact dressing* (e.g. Mepitel) and an absorbent pad (e.g. Foam).

Protection of the surrounding skin is paramount to prevent further breakdown of the wound. A protective *non-alcohol skin barrier film* (e.g. Cavilon) is recommended.

For fungating wounds that are discrete with intact surrounding skin, the use of a small *stoma appliance* might be useful. For larger exuding wounds, a *wound manager* appliance that allows close monitoring and visibility of the wound may be applied.[16]

Malodour

One of the most distressing symptoms for a patient with a fungating wound is malodour.[17] The removal of necrotic tissue which can provide a growth medium for bacteria to thrive may be useful in preventing infection. If infection is already present, appropriate antibiotics should be commenced, taking into account any potential side effects these may cause.

The characteristic smell that is associated with malignant fungating wounds is due to anaerobic organisms that flourish in the accessible necrotic tissue. These organisms produce volatile fatty acids as an end-product, which are particularly offensive.[15]

The aims of management are (see Table 8.2):

- to debride the necrotic tissue
- to kill the anaerobic organisms
- to filter out and control the odour.

Table 8.2 Malodour reference table

No exudate	Exudate present
Good ventilation	Good ventilation
Systemic metronidazole	Systemic metronidazole
Metronidazole gel (0.8–0.9%)	Charcoal and hydrofibre dressing
Charcoal dressings	
Honey	
Sugar paste	
Larval therapy (may produce exudates)	

Metronidazole gel (0.8–0.9%) is an effective debriding agent. It works by killing the bacteria responsible for the odour production and it can be safely mixed with other gels (e.g. hydrogels) in order to facilitate debridement. Use is recommended for 5–7 days, but this may be repeated to keep odour under control.[18,19]

Systemic metronidazole should be used with caution because of the known side effects especially in this group of patients who may be heavily dependent on alcohol. Sparrow *et al.*[20] demonstrated that metronidazole could be used in lower doses of 200 mg three times a day with effectiveness and fewer side effects.

Activated charcoal dressings (can be combined with silver) attract and bind the molecules which cause the odour and thus prevent their escape from the local area.[21] An example of this dressing is Clinisorb. Silver is released from the dressing and exerts an antibacterial activity (e.g. Aquacel Ag, Acticoat).

Charcoal dressings become ineffective if they become wet,[12] so caution is advised, especially with head and neck wounds that often develop sinuses and/or fistulae with profuse amounts of exudates. A combined charcoal and hydrofibre dressing may be useful in these circumstances (e.g Carboflex).

Sugar paste can be useful in debriding wounds and sometimes aids regranulation.[22] It is available commercially from Northwest London Hospitals NHS Trust (Pharmacy, Northwick Park Hospital) in thick and thin preparations. Twice daily dressings are recommended.[21]

Honey has regained popularity recently. Antibacterial activity results from the presence of small quantities of hydrogen peroxide which is an oxidizing agent released by the action of the enzyme peroxidase that is added by bees to the nectar they collect.[23] Some honey has plant-derived antibacterial properties which have an anti-inflammatory effect, although this can be destroyed by heat. If the honey comes into contact with excessive exudates, this will cause dilution and therefore render the honey ineffective.[24]

Gamma-irradiated honey is recommended as this has been correctly sterilized and will not cause any infection control issues.[24] Honey is now available on the Drug Tariff in impregnated sheet preparations (e.g. Activon Tulle; Medihoney).

Larval therapy is sometimes used for rapid debridment. Their mode of action is to move over the surface of the wound, secreting a powerful mixture of proteolytic enzymes which break down dead tissue and liquidize it. It can result in a significant increase in exudate production of which the patient should be informed. This therapy should not be used on wounds that contain fistulae or that are connected to vital organs.[25] Patient compliance is an important issue. Careful counselling and information is required.

Other strategies include the use of environmental air filters, good ventilation, and essential oils, although these should be used with care as they can add to the pungent odour.[10]

The psychological impact for the patient who has a malodorous wound can never be under estimated. These issues will be dealt with in the section 'Psychological issues'.

Pain

Pain can be experienced locally as well as generalized pain from the tumour and/or metastatic disease.

Pain is caused by:

- pressure on nerves and blood vessels
- exposure of the dermis and associated nerve endings
- surrounding oedema and/or excoriated skin
- trauma to the wound during dressing changes.[16,26]
  Ongoing pain assessment is vital.

> The patient's description of the type and severity of pain must be accepted as true. Pain is always subjective and patients' pain is what they say it is and not what others think it ought to be (Woodruff[27]).

Assessment should be regularly undertaken using an evidence-based tool that is effective and user friendly.[4,28] In the author's Trust, a complex wound assessment tool has been devised, which provides visual analogue scales for pain, malodour, and exudate. Assessment tools can be useful if they are used by trained health care professionals in conjunction with patients.

Non-pharmacological interventions

- Warm saline 0.9% for cleansing.
- Care whilst removing dressings.
- Maintain a moist environment at wound bed.
- Avoid toxic substances (e.g. iodine).

Wound dressing should be selected according to wound requirements and needs. Adhesives should be avoided if the surrounding skin is fragile. *Silicone dressings* are useful as they are non-adherent and easy to remove.[2,27]

Pharmacological interventions

- Opioids—regular analgesia should continue in order to treat the patient's baseline pain. The use of breakthrough analgesia can be incorporated for dressing changes.[10]
- Non-steroidal anti-inflammatory drugs and neuropathic agents may also be effective in treating associated wound pain.[28]
- Short-acting measures (e.g. Entonox) can be useful if dressing changes are particularly painful.[29]
- Lidocaine gel can provide some relief, but patients may complain of stinging.
- Topical opioids—there is some evidence that there are opioid receptors present in peripheral nerves.[28,30] These receptors become active when inflammation occurs. Several case reports have reported satisfactory results using opioids mixed with a hydrogel and applied directly to the wound. Different opioids have been used: diamorphine;[31] morphine;[32] and fentanyl.[33] When pain at the wound site is a particular problem, it is worth trying topical opioids and evaluating the effect for 48 h.

Suggested prescription (from author's personal experience):

Morphine for injection 10–20 mg once or twice daily

mixed with

Hydrogel 15–30 g once or twice daily (can use metronidazole gel)

If the wound covers a vast amount of skin (e.g. chest wall disease) and the patient complains of pain at the wound site, it is imperative that a full

Case study

A 43-year-old gentleman had a neurofibromatosis of his left buttock. This had spread locally over his right buttock, down both thighs to mid thigh, and up over his lower back region. The wound was enormous and difficult to dress. The patient complained of intense pain at the wound site, during and after dressings. On assessment, it was evident that the pain was isolated to a small area approximately 8 cm × 5.5 cm. Topical opioids were applied to this area only with excellent effect.

assessment of the wound expanse is conducted. It is not advisable to apply topical opioids liberally to the entire wound as systemic uptake is unknown. In the author's experience, there may be isolated areas where the pain is more prominent and the topical opioids can be applied to this area only.

Pruritis

This may occur around the margin of the wound. A gentle *moisturizing cream* (e.g. aqueous cream with menthol) may be applied, and care should be taken not to use adhesives that will cause further irritation.

Cavilon—a *non-alcohol skin barrier film* provides additional protection from exudates which can exacerbate pruritis.

Lidocaine gel can also be applied to the surrounding area.

Bleeding

Bleeding may occur in the fragile and friable vasculature due to tumour activity. It can also be related to the application of inappropriate dressings. Careful selection of dressings can be instrumental in the prevention of bleeding. A decreased platelet count (due to anticancer treatment) may also exacerbate the bleeding.

Certain *alginates* (e.g. Kaltostat) have been said to provide haemostatic properties, but care should be taken in the use of these as minimal exudates can result in the fibres of the dressing becoming intertwined in the wound and cause additional trauma and bleeding on removal.[2]

Topical applications

- Adrenaline 1:1000—gauze soak to wound and pressure applied. There is a risk of ischaemic necrosis due to local vasoconstriction.[2] This should not be applied regularly as little is known regarding systemic uptake.

- Tranexamic acid—at 1–1.5 g twice to four times a day orally or the via feeding tube for prevention of bleeding.[34] This can also be applied topically using the injection preparation.
- Sucralfate—paste or suspension applied directly to the wound.[35]
- Haemostatic surgical sponges (e.g. Spongostan). These dressings are very useful in controlling fast bleeds. Unfortunately, these are very difficult for community staff to access (expensive and not available on the Drug Tariff) but are beneficial to have if the patient is at risk of a bleed.[2]

Securing dressings

Finding a method of securing appropriate dressings to a wound in this population of patients is extremely challenging. Frequently the skin surrounding the wound is too fragile to use tape, and facial hair can cause problems with adhesion.

Tapeless retention dressings are available which are hypoallergenic and easy to use,[36] but these can be expensive and there are concerns about infection control with repeated use.

Netelast may be useful for lower head and neck areas.

Involving the patient in the quest to find a way to secure the dressing is paramount, and often they will initiate ideas whilst working alongside the health care professional. Patients often welcome being involved and can contribute valuable suggestions. In such a visible area, patient acceptance is an important element of the dressing process and nursing care. Disguising the dressings with scarves and hats may also be useful.

Innovation and imagination are the key concepts for this area of care as there is no clear answer to this problem.

Fistulae

Oro-cutaneous fistulae following flap repair and/or breakdown of a wound occurs in approximately 4% of patients.[37] Drainage from fistulae can be profuse and can result in infection, excoriation, and odour.

If possible, a stoma appliance bag should be applied to a draining fistula. This avoids repeated dressings and allows for protection of the surrounding skin. Before a stoma bag is secured in position, the application of a barrier film (e.g. Cavilon) should be used to the surrounding skin.

Advice from the stoma specialist nurse should be sought.

Psychological issues

For the patient with a fungating wound, the visual reminder of their cancer is always present,[38–40] as well as the added burden of disease progression and impending death.[41,42]

It is frequently mentioned that each fungating wound is unique to the individual, and management should reflect this.[9] The impact on the family is also noted,[8] and that this should be taken into consideration when planning the patient's care.

There is reference made to the challenging and difficult nature of these wounds and their possible impact on the patient's life. Van Toller[43] suggested that patients afflicted by malodour would be sure to lose quality of life and this may take the form of withdrawal, depression, and a reluctance to engage in any social activities. Piggin[44] also acknowledges the importance of considering the wider impact of malodorous wounds for the patient, and comments on the associated social values and stigma.

Research conducted by the author for her MSc dissertation focused on gaining an understanding of the views, perceptions, and impact on the life of an individual with a fungating malignant wound.[40] Interviews with patients with fungating malignant wounds revealed that they felt they were on an *emotional and psychological rollercoaster* (Fig. 8.4). The emotions are similar to a fairground ride. Patients felt relief and joy when they reached a plateau when their wound and disease were stable. They were riding high on adrenaline and never knew what would happen next. There was pleasure and excitement mixed with worry and anxiety in case something else went

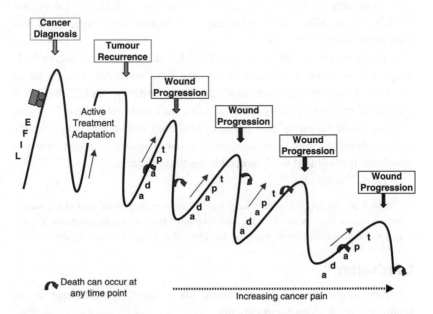

Fig 8.4 The rollercoaster ride. Living with a fungating malignant wound.

Case report

Douglas was a 54-year-old gentleman with a synovial sarcoma of his left leg. His favourite pastime was dancing, and he and his long-term partner belonged to a club, which they went to 3–4 evenings a week. Since his diagnosis, his passion for dancing grew. He felt that he was 'normal' and 'alive' when he could dance, and he 'measured' how his wound was by his ability to dance. For him, it was 'good' if he could dance without the wound leaking or smelling, but it was 'bad' if the tumour was active and the wound was progressing—enlarging and causing symptoms. He described the joy he felt when he could dance and the 'absolute depression' when he had to sit and watch.

wrong. Inevitably the peak fell away when the disease and wound progressed and they were left tumbling down, emotionally and physically.

Patients also talked about being a burden on their carers and how they tried to protect them from any bad news so that they would remain strong. They referred to going through a continuous cycle of adaptation and readjustment which was especially difficult if they had children. Patients acknowledged that it was not always possible to adapt, and it may be haphazard and unpredictable, depending on their own personal expectations. This theme was evident in their coping skills and them finding strength from other sources such as their social support network

Lastly, they referred to 'covering up', which related to their altered body image and society's reactions to them. The head and neck patients talked about their need to rearrange their lifestyle in order to 'fit in'. They often 'bracketed' themselves off by avoiding pertinent issues and society.

The issues of 'normalcy' and 'taking control' were important throughout the themes identified, but these elements battled against the uncertainty and emotional turmoil that was predictable for these patients.

As Doyle[45] aptly says:

Can we begin to imagine what it must feel like for a patient to see part of his body rotting and to have to live with the offensive smell from it, see the reactions of his visitors (including doctors and nurses) and know that it signifies lingering death?

Conclusion

Complex fungating, malignant wounds are a significant challenge for all health care professionals and patients.

Holistic assessment is paramount because it focuses on caring for the patient as a complete being and not the wound in isolation.

As health care professionals we should aim to:

- be aware of the aim(s) of the treatment at all times
- be realistic about the aims—and discuss them with the patient
- remember that each wound is unique and will mean something different to each patient
- establish a cohesive and open relationship with the patient
- provide adequate and timely assessment
- use clear, rational decision making regarding symptom control measures
- always use skilful communication
- demonstrate tact, understanding, and supportive care.

Much can be done to keep the lesions comfortable and odourless but the attitude with which the dressing is performed will do more to alleviate the patient's feelings of shame, disgust and alienation than any of the many potions (Charles-Edwards[46]).

References

1 Moody, M., and Grocott, P. (1993). Let us extend our knowledge base: assessment and management of fungating malignant wounds. *Prof Nurse*, **8**, 587–589.

2 Grocott, P. (2000). Palliative management of fungating malignant wounds. *J Community Nurs*, **14**, 31–40.

3 Mera, S. (1997). *Pathology and understanding disease prevention*. Cheltenham, UK, Stanley, Thomas.

4 Grocott, P. (2001). *The palliative management of fungating malignant wounds*. Wound Care Educational Booklet; 8, 2.

5 Thomas, S. (1992). *Current practices in the management of fungating lesions and radiation damaged skin*. Bridgend, UK, Surgical Materials Testing Laboratories.

6 Schwartz, R.A. (1995). Cutaneous metastatic disease. *J Am Acad Dermatol*, **33**, 161–182.

7 Laverty, D., Mallett, J., and Mulholland, J. (1997). Protocols and guidelines for managing wounds. *Prof Nurse*, **13**, 79–81.

8 Naylor, W., Laverty, D., and Mallett, J. (2001). *The Royal Marsden Hospital handbook of wound management in cancer care*. Oxford, Blackwell Science.

9 Haisfield-Wolfe, M.E., and Rund, C. (1997). Malignant cutaneous wounds: a management protocol. *Ostomy/Wound Manag*, **43**, 56–66.

10 Naylor, W., Laverty, D., and Soady, C. (2004). *The Royal Marsden Hospital manual of clinical nursing procedures*, 6th edn. Oxford. Blackwell Science.

11 Grocott, P. (1995). The palliative management of fungating malignant wounds. *J Wound Care*, **4**, 240–242.

12 Collier, M. (2000). Management of patients with fungating wounds. *Nurs Stand*, **15**, 46–52.

13 Gould, D. (1999). Wound management and pain control. *Nurs Stand*, **14**, 47–54.

14 Gilchrist, B. (1999). Wound infection. In Miller, M. and Glover, D., eds. *Wound management theory and practice*, pp. 96–107. London, Nursing Times Books.

15 Grocott, P. (1999). The management of fungating wounds. *J Wound Care*, **8**, 232–234.

16 Wilson, V. (2005) Assessment and management of fungating wounds: a review. *Wound Care*, March, S28–S34.

17 Benbow, M. (1999). Malodorous wounds: how to improve quality of life. *Community Nurse*, **5**, 43–46.

18 Finlay, I,G., Bowszyc, J., Ramlav, C., and Gwiezdzinski, Z. (1996). The effect of topical 0.75% metronidazole on malodorous cutaneous ulcers. *J Pain Sympt Manag*, **11**, 158–162.

19 Moody, M. (2001). Metrotop: a topical antimicrobial agent for malodorous wounds. *Br J Nurs*, **7**, 286–289.

20 Sparrow, G., Minton, M., Rubens, R.D., Simmons, N.A., and Aubrey, C. (1980). Metronidazole in smelly tumours. *Lancet*, **i**, 1185.

21 Thomas, S., Fischer, B., Fram, P.J., *et al.* (1998). Odour absorbing dressings. *J Wound Care*, **7**, 246–250.

22 Topham, J. (2000). Sugar for wounds. *J Tissue Viability*, **10**, 86–89.

23 Kinsley, A. (2001). A proactive approach to wound infection. *Nurs Stand*, **15**, 50–58.

24 Dunford, C., Cooper, R., Molan, P., and White, R. (2000). The use of honey on wound management. *Nurs Stand*, **15**, 63–68.

25 Thomas, S., Jones, M., Wynn, K., and Fowler, T. (2001). The current status of maggot therapy in wound healing. *Br J Nurs*, **10**, Suppl 5–12.

26 Manning, M.P. (1998). Metastasis to skin. *Semin Oncol Nurs*, **14**, 240–243.

27 Woodruff, R. (1997). *Cancer pain*. Melbourne, Asperula Pty Ltd.

28 Naylor, W. (2002). Symptom self-assessment in the management of fungating wounds. http://www.worldwidewounds.com/2002/july/Naylor.Part2/Wound.Assessment.-Tool.html Accessed July 12, 2005.

29 Collier, M., and Hollinworth, H. (2000). Pain and tissue trauma at the time of dressing changes. *Nurs Stand*, **14**, 71–73.

30 Naylor, W. (2001). Assessment and management of pain in fungating wounds. *Br J Nurs*, **10**, Suppl 33–52.

31 Hollinworth, H. (1997). Less pain, more gain. *Nurs Times*, **93**, 89–91.

32 Krajnik, M., Zylicz, Z., Finlay, I., Luczak, J., and van Sorge, A.A. (1999). Potential uses of topical opioids in palliative care: report of 6 cases. *Pain*, **80**, 121–125.

33 Back, I., and Finlay, I. (1995). Analgesic effect of topical opioids on painful skin ulcers. *J Pain Symptom Manag*, **10**, 493.

34 Krajnik, M., and Zylicz, Z. (1997). Topical morphine for the cutaneous cancer pain. *Palliative Med*, **11**, 325.

35 Paul, J.R. (2000). Analgesia of painful skin ulcers with topical gel containing fentanyl citrate—four case reports (Research Abstracts). *Palliative Med*, **14**, 335.

36 Dean, A. (1997). Fibrinolytic inhibitors for cancer associated bleeding problems. *J Pain Sympt Control*, **13**, 20–24.

37 Emflorgo, C. (1998). Controlling bleeding in fungating wounds (Letter). *J Wound Care*, **7**, 235.

38 McGregor, F., and Baxter, H. (1999). Staying power. *Nurs Times*, **95**, 66–71.

39 O'Brien, C.J., Lee, K.K., Stern, H.S., *et al.* (1998). Evaluation of 250 free flap recon-structions after resection of tumours of the head and neck. *Aust NZ J Surg*, **68**, 698–701.

40 Price, E. (1996). The stigma of smell. *Nursing Times*, **92**(20); 70–73.

41 Wilkes, L., Boxer, E., and White, K. (2003). The hidden side of nursing: why caring for patients with malignant malodorous wounds is so difficult. *J Wound Care*, **12**, 76–80.

42 Laverty, D. (2004). A rollercoaster ride: living with a fungating, malignant wound. MSc Dissertation, RCN Institute.

43 Pudner, R. (1998). The management of patients with a fungating or malignant wound. *J Community Nurs*, **12**, 1–6.

44 Bird, C. (2000). Managing malignant fungating wounds. *Prof Nurse*, **15**, 253–256.

45 Van Toller, S. (1994). Invisible wounds: the effects of skin ulcer malodours. *J Wound Care*, **3**, 103–105.

46 Piggin, C. (2003). Malodorous fungating wounds: uncertain concepts underlying the management of social isolation. *Int J Palliative Nurs*, **9**, 216–221.

47 Doyle, D. (1980). Domicillary terminal care. *The Practitioner*, **224**, 575–582.

48 Charles-Edwards, A. (1983). *The nursing care of the dying patient.* Beaconsfield, UK, Beaconsfield Publishers.

Chapter 9

Pain management in advanced and recurrent disease

Marc Webster and Neil A. Hagen

Introduction

Head and neck cancers share several features with other solid tumours: they have become increasingly prevalent over the past few decades, in keeping with increasing tobacco use in the 1960s and 1970s; they are treated with a combination of radical surgery, radical radiotherapy, and cytotoxic chemo-therapy; and early diagnosis can increase the likelihood of successful treat-ment. Distinct from other cancer types, patients with head and neck cancer who develop progressive disease are at particular risk of difficulty controlling secretions and obtaining adequate nutrition, and of developing respiratory distress. Also, pain can be difficult to manage owing to a variety of specific characteristics. However, the knowledge, skills, and attitudes central to a palliative approach to head and neck cancers can be particularly helpful to improve quality of life and maintain dignity, and it is to that end that this chapter is focused. This chapter will outline the epidemiology of pain in the head and neck patient, review salient features of the history and physical examination, and outline the pathophysiology of pain. Specific pain syn-dromes will be reviewed, including those due to cancer treatment (such as mucositis and post-surgical neuropathic pain) and those directly due to cancer. Finally, an overall management strategy for pain in patients with head and neck malignancies will be presented, including non-drug, drug, and invasive analgesic interventions.

Epidemiology

A large proportion of head and neck cancer patients (40–80%) will experience pain during the course of their illness. Pain can be the manifestation which heralds the diagnosis of the cancer, it can appear during treatment, post-therapy, or at recurrence. In a prospective study by Chaplin and colleagues, 93 patients were followed longitudinally, and pain was the first symptom of cancer in half of the participants.[1] Treatment-related pain is also a prominent problem in the patient with head and neck cancer.

The interventions used to treat the cancer influence the likelihood of developing pain. Combined modality therapy using concurrent chemoradiotherapy results in nearly universal, severe, but transient mucositis. Mucositis can greatly affect quality of life, through pain and impaired ability to perform basic life functions such as eating and swallowing. Combined modality treatment is also associated with a high risk of *chronic* therapy-related pain: Wilgen and colleagues examined 153 patients 1 year post-operatively and found that 33% reported neck pain, with a neuropathic component in almost all affected individuals (hyperpathia, i.e. pinprick felt to be too sharp, in 96%; and allodynia, i.e. light touch of the skin results in pain, in 39%). In this study, administration of radiotherapy was a significant contributing factor.[2]

Finally, pain was a common sign of recurrent disease, described by 70% of 95 patients. This high prevalence of pain is thought to be because recurrence is most common in the well innervated oropharyngeal and nasopharyngeal areas;[3] pain may be less common in hypopharyngeal sites of recurrence presumably on the basis of relatively less innervation in this region.

However, many studies of the epidemiology of pain in head and neck cancer patients are small, underpowered, and subject to a variety of biases; further work remains to be done in the epidemiology of symptoms associated with head and neck cancers and their treatment.

Quality of life

There has been a shift in focus in clinical trials and in the overall practice of medical oncology. In the past, the emphasis was on traditional primary treatment outcomes such as overall survival, disease-free survival, response rate, and so on. More recently, there is attention paid to the impact of cancer therapy on health-related quality of life. Indeed, functional and physical impairments coupled with potential negative influences on social and psychological well-being have a major influence on the head and neck cancer patient. Unfortunately health-related quality of life assessment has been poorly studied in the past and only now are we exploring the full impact of treatment experienced by the patient. Further, there is great variability of symptoms depending on the site of malignancy (nasopharyngeal vs. oropharynx vs. oral cavity vs. larynx), treatment modality (sugery, radiotherapy, both surgery and radiotherapy, chemo-radiotherapy, and so on), and lack of concordance seen with the several available validated quality of life assessment tools. In general, primary surgery can greatly affect function and personal well-being, through disfigurement, dysphonia (or aphonia), dysphagia, drooling, respiratory difficulties, and loss or distorted sense of smell. Radiotherapy can cause difficulty with swallowing and chewing, xerostomia (dry mouth), dysphagia, osteoradionecrosis (ORN), stricture, temporomandibular joint dysfunction, and neck contractures, to list a few. Although no randomized controlled trials have specifically compared the impact on long-term quality of life with radiotherapy compared with surgery, studies tend to support radiotherapy with or without chemotherapy as having better quality of life in the long term compared with surgery alone.[4,5] Improved pain-related scores were observed in the VA larynx study comparing surgery vs. combined chemotherapy/radiotherapy in laryngeal cancers.[6]

Overall, however, quality of life is often poor in patients with head and neck cancer. In a prospective, multi-institutional study following 357 patients with head and neck cancer, overall health-related quality of life fell during treatment, with gradual return to baseline by 12 months. Pharyngeal site of the primary and advanced stage were the factors most closely correlated with worse scores.[7] Older age, low socio-economic status, advanced malignancy, and flap reconstruction are other factors that predict poor health-related quality of life in head and neck cancer patients.[8]

Barriers to effective pain management

Cancer pain can be effectively managed in the large majority of cancer patients through an integrated approach using both pharmacological and non-pharmacological therapies. Patients with more difficult pain problems may benefit from a variety of interventional approaches. Intractable pain remains a common concern for cancer patients. Unfortunately, despite the impressive overall success rate in managing pain, several barriers exist[9] and in particular there is a need for improved professional education, principally within medical and nursing professions. A disproportionately small percentage of time is devoted to pain and symptom management issues within undergraduate and postgraduate training curriculae given the high prevalence of pain within the cancer population. Further, the complexity of the pathophysiological mechanisms of pain and complexities of available pharmacological interventions can pose barriers to successful outcomes. An evidence-based approach to patient assessment and management will be greatly supported by further clinical research in this area. Patient concerns about the risks of opioids, public misunderstanding about pain, and lack of support for patient and family coping skills provide additional barriers in better managing pain in head and neck cancer patients.

Pain history, physical examination, and investigations

The pain history and physical exam are essential to formulate the differential diagnosis and construct an individualized intervention strategy. However, the stakes are high: since half of patients with head and neck cancer present with pain as an early manifestation, a herald of the diagnosis, bed-side assessment, if performed expertly, can facilitate identification of an early, potentially curable local tumour.

Whether the cancer is at an early or advanced stage, there are several key components of the pain history. These include a description of prominent characteristics of the pain: aggravating and relieving factors, radiation of pain, duration, intensity, analgesic interventions, and their outcomes. Pain scales are useful tools to document effectiveness of analgesic interventions, such as a numerical pain score, with '0' being 'no pain' and '10' being 'the worst possible pain'. Evaluation to assess for delirium, depression, anxiety, or other treatable affective disorders should be undertaken as needed. Finally, no treatment plan can be formulated without knowledge of the patient's goals and expectations. Patients need to understand the status of their underlying disease and ultimate prognosis.

Descriptors of pain are commonly used to guide the clinician to discerning the underlying broad mechanism of pain—somatic, visceral, or neuropathic. *Neuropathic pain* is often described as burning, pins and needles, numbness, or a crawling sensation; and can be paroxysmal (sudden and brief) or continuous. Commonly used terms to characterize neuropathic pain include *allodynia* (pain from an innocuous stimulus such as light touch), *hyperalgesia* (abnormal severity of pain from noxious stimuli, such as a gentle touch by a pin being experienced as painfully sharp), and *neuralgia* (brief, stabbing, and often electrical pain, felt along the distribution of a nerve). *Visceral pain* is typically dull, crampy, poorly localized, and is often referred (e.g. diaphragmatic irritation manifest as ipsilateral shoulder pain) while *somatic pain* can be sharp or dull but is usually well localized. When somatic, visceral, or neuropathic pain occur together, the term '*mixed pain*' is used. Each contributes to the overall pain experience, thereby making treatment decisions more complex; not surprisingly, mixed pain carries a less good overall prognosis for successful management.

The physical examination of the head and neck cancer patient with pain begins with a general physical exam, to evaluate the extent of the malignancy and evaluate for co-morbidity such as peripheral vascular disease, lung disease, poor dentition, or other conditions that can impact pain management. Next the clinician should focus on the region of the pain. Ask the patient, 'show me, where exactly do you hurt?' Inspect, looking for evidence of infection, tumour, or other evident pathology. Very gently palpate the area, looking for allodynia (see above), or soft tissue or other tenderness. Evaluate for evidence of cancer, including an intraoral exam. Next, systematically palpate, move, and in other ways gently stress potentially pain-sensitive structures. In the head and neck region, for example, this will include palpation of muscles (looking for myofascial pain), bones, ligaments, arteries, and other tissues. Then undertake range of motion of the neck in six directions: flexion; extension; left and right lateral flexion; and left and right lateral rotation. The goal is to identify all possible sources of the pain.[10]

After completing the general and the regional physical examination, formulate the pain diagnosis. Is the pain somatic, visceral, neuropathic, or mixed? What is the most likely pain-sensitive structure? Is the mechanism due to tumour, infection, treatment-related pain? Note that *treatment-related* pain only rarely occurs out of the blue, months after treatment has been completed; recurrent cancer is a much more likely cause.

Consider if diagnostic investigations could help rule in or rule out the hypothesis you have generated from findings on the history and physical examination. Serum electrolytes can help assess underlying treatable causes of delirium, while culture of infected areas can identify appropriate targeted antimicrobial therapy. Imaging is often required to confirm underlying pathology contributing to the pain and to document stage, thereby informing prognosis and decisions on potential disease-modifying strategies. Computed tomography (CT) has established itself as the modality of choice in baseline work-up of the newly diagnosed head and neck cancer patient, although magnetic resonance imaging (MRI) and more recently positron emission tomography (PET) scanning have complementary roles in assessing soft tissue masses and recurrent disease, respectively.[11] MRI is less helpful in the previously treated patient due to tissue distortion from surgery and post-radiotherapy scarring.

Pathophysiology—mechanisms of pain

The pain experience is remarkably individual. The neurophysiology of pain includes peripheral mechanisms and central mechanisms. Each step of this process involves several layers of control that can increase, perpetuate, or reduce it.

In the periphery, physical, chemical, or other stimuli can cause action potentials to be developed by pain receptors ('nociceptors'). The stimuli that can result in pain signals being generated in the periphery are many, including ischaemia, tissue injury, inflammation, infection, and stretch. Nociceptors are primarily associated with small, unmyelinated C fibres. However, polymodal receptors respond to a variety of other stimuli but can generate painful sensations under specific circumstances such as tissue injury. Once stimulated, the nociceptive signal is propagated along the A-delta or C-fibres to the dorsal horn of the spinal cord where they synapse with second-order nociceptive neurons. Second-order neurons cross to the contralateral side of the spinal cord and ascend upward to the thalamus where pain is first perceived. They also project to various subcortical structures including the periaqueductal grey and reticular formation, and hypothalamus. After synapsing, the third-order neurons project from the thalamus to every lobe of the brain, with only about 40% of pain information going to the cortical sensory strip where pain is more accurately localized.

Descending analgesic pathways modulate incoming nociceptive (pain) information. Numerous interconnections between structures important in the awareness of pain and for modulation of the pain stimulus result in the wide range of personal perception of pain to seemingly identical initial stimuli.

Pain has several common causes in head and neck cancer patients. Specific syndromes are related to cancer treatment, such as oral mucositis and ORN. Cranial neuralgias are particularly common in head and neck cancer patients. Also common are focal syndromes directly related to cancer invasion of specific structures such as base of skull metastases.

Treatment-related pain

Mucositis

Perhaps the most prevalent of pain syndromes in the head and neck cancer population is that experienced during treatment—mucositis associated with radiotherapy, chemotherapy, or both. This represents a highly challenging clinical problem as it is associated with transient but severe disability and, at times, can be life threatening.

Normally the oral mucosa undergoes renewal over a 7–14 day cycle. The effects of radiation or chemotherapy treatment on the oral mucosa therefore become most symptomatic 1–2 weeks following treatment.[12,13] While all oral mucosa is susceptible, there is a predilection for increased damage to poorly keratinized tissue (relatively sparing the lips and oesophagus). The severity of pain and mucositis experienced by patients is dependent on several factors, including concurrent infection, use of medications, xerostomia (and there are several mechanisms of dry mouth following treatment of head and neck cancer), type of chemotherapy, underlying performance status, nutritional status, and overall immune status. Effective management of mucositis and its exacerbating factors represents an important part of the overall acumen needed for care of head and neck cancer patients.

Medications

Medications can play a significant role in maintaining or worsening the mucosal damage associated with radiotherapy and chemotherapy. Indeed opioids, which are a cornerstone of symptom management, can worsen xerostomia thereby exacerbating stomatitis and pain.[14] The use of adjuvant analgesics and early diagnosis of secondary infections can minimize the negative impact of the use of opioids. Other medications typically implicated in dry mouth include those with strong anticholinergic properties (antispasmotics, certain tricyclic antidepressants, antidiarrhoeal agents, antiemetics, antihistamines, and certain neuroleptics), in addition to various antihypertensives, diuretics and sedatives.[15] Being alert to the potential effect of these medications and their judicious use may aid in both recovery from and reduction in the severity of the mucositis.

Infections

The normal protective oral mucosa can be damaged from both direct and indirect effects of therapy. Also, the immune system is often impaired from chemotherapy and transient malnutrition (from odynophagia and anorexia). Thus head and neck cancer patients are predisposed to a variety of infections that complicate mucositis.[16,17] Local infection activates inflammatory cells which secrete cytokines and prostaglandins, both of which stimulate nociceptors, and these at least partially account for the increased pain and aggravation of the underlying stomatitis. With the development of sudden worsening of stomatitis symptoms, one should look for evidence of a coincidental infection particularly in the immunocompromised patient.

Bacterial When the serum neutrophil count drops below $1 \times 10^9/l$, the likelihood of bacterial infection increases substantially. This is commonly seen with the use of myelosuppressive chemotherapeutics. Cisplatin in combination with 5-fluorouracil—a common chemotherapy regimen in head and neck cancers—typically produces grade 3–4 haematological toxicities in up to four-fifths of patients.[18,19] The development of fever in a neutropenic patient is a life-threatening scenario requiring comprehensive evaluation and administration of intravenous antibiotics. Strong consideration should be given to including vancomycin in the initial antibiotic regimen in head and neck cancer patients, given the preponderance of Gram-positive organisms (especially *Streptococcus viridans*) in these circumstances.[20]

Fungal and viral Even with normal white blood cell (WBC) counts, both fungal and viral infections are commonly seen during treatment of head and neck cancers. Candidal infections are reported with the greatest frequency, ranging from 20 and 50% of all patients with mucositis.[21,17] This may even underestimate the true prevalence given the difficulty in differentiating the atrophic form of this infection from radiation-induced ulceration. Treatment typically uses antifungal agents, with nystatin and fluconazole being the most frequently prescribed. Fluconazole has both clinical and microbiological superiority over nystatin,[22,23] making it the drug of choice; however, higher cost limits its universal use as first-line therapy.

Herpes simplex reactivation and infection is another cause of painful stomatitis (inflammation of the oral mucosa). It is clearly described in patients who have undergone bone marrow or solid organ transplant, where there is evidence that routine prophylaxis should be used. However, the role of prophylaxis of herpes infections in head and neck patients receiving radiotherapy or combined modality treatment is a subject of ongoing study. Eptein *et al.* examined 19 herpes-seropositive patients receiving radiotherapy alone and demonstrated positive cultures in four patients.[24] Likewise, Nicelatou isolated herpes simples virus 1 (HSV-1) from ulcers in five of 14 patients.[25] Conflicting data from others have not shown such high reactivation rates or effects on mucositis;[26,27] however, all studies to date are small or do not analyse the impact of combined chemo-radiotherapy on the risk of reactivation. Regardless, reactivation of herpes can cause significant morbidity in the acute exacerbation of mucositis.[28] Viral infections typically involve the keratinized mucosa of the gingiva, hard palate, and dorsum of the tongue. The presentation is often difficult or impossible to differentiate from ulceration induced by radiotherapy. Acyclovir and related compounds are effective in reducing the burden of established disease, often anecdotally resulting in significant pain relief.[25] Early antiviral institution also limits the establishment or degree of post-HSV-1 neuralgia. Given the controversy surrounding the impact of HSV reactivation in treating head and neck malignancies, antiviral prophylaxis is not routinely recommended; however, further research in this area is warranted.

Prevention and limiting the extent of mucositis

Prophylactic and ongoing mouth care is helpful to reduce complications from mucositis.[29] This includes routine pre-treatment dental consultation; saline or soda rinses during treatment; removable prostheses; and avoidance of oral irritants such as alcohol, smoking, and spicy foods. Many different interventions have aimed at minimizing the severity and high frequency of mucositis encountered with current treatment regimens. A detailed discussion of specific treatments for mucositis is beyond the scope of this review; however, a brief overview will be presented with focus on radiation- or chemoradiation-induced mucositis. The reader may wish to consult recent publications on this topic.[30–32]

Amifostine

Amifostine or WR-1065 was initially designed as a radioprotectant for soldiers in the event of potential radiation exposure. It is an organic thiophosphate which is dephosphorylated in tissues to its active metabolite which functions as a free radical scavenger. The dephosphorylating enzyme responsible for activation is found in greater quantity in normal vs. malignant tissues, allowing selectivity without compromising antitumour effects.[33] While many studies have examined the mucositis-sparing effect of amifostine, the largest randomized controlled trial has demonstrated only a trend toward improvement.[34] Given the heterogeneity seen in currently published trials in route of administration, dose, and concomitant antitumour treatments, this obscures any conclusive benefit which may exist. Despite the equivocal results in reducing the severity of acute mucositis, its use has been firmly established to reduce development of chronic xerostomia.[35]

Oral cryotherapy

Oral cryotherapy is an attempt to limit access of chemotherapy to oral mucosa through reactive vasoconstriction induced by local cooling methods. It has been shown to reduce statistically the severity of mucositis with 5-fluorouracil-containing regimens.[36] Given the tumour's proximity to the oral mucosa in some patients, a reduction in blood flow and, in theory, decreased delivery of the chemosensitizing drug would negate any intended therapeutic effects and therefore cannot be recommended.

Prophylactic antibiotic decontamination

Several studies have examined the benefit of prophylactic antibiotic pastilles to reduce the microbial load, in the hope of preventing the contributing effects of mucosal infection to mucositis. Here again results are mixed. Okuno et al. found no difference in mucositis scores,[37] while Symonds noted reduced dysphagia and weight loss in the active treatment group.[38] Although the evidence supporting the use of prophylactic antibiotics is mixed at present, the use of the broad-spectrum topical antimicrobial chlorhexidine has consistently shown inferior results and is potentially harmful.[39] Its use should be avoided.

Anti-inflammatory agents

As a topical anti-inflammatory agent, benzydamine has shown promise in reducing the severity and duration of mucositis in several studies.[40–42] Pentoxifylline, a xanthine derivative, is capable of downregulating tumour necrosis factor-α (TNF-α) and in preclinical data shown to reduce endotoxin caused by radiation damage. While no study has been reported for its use in head and neck malignancies, variable results have been achieved in the setting of high dose chemotherapy with stem cell transplant patients.[43,44]

Barrier agents

Sucralfate is a non-absorbable aluminium salt capable of adhering to ulcer bases, creating a protective coating. It enjoyed much attention in early studies, only to be found ineffective in larger double-blinded studies.[45,46] A bioadherent oral gel containing polyvinylpyrollidone and hyaluronate (Gelclair) is being studied in various patient populations with mucositis and is showing some promise.[47] Its use in the head and neck cancer population is unstudied but this would clearly be an obvious target population in which to test its efficacy.

Topical analgesia

In an attempt to limit systemic opioid requirements, various mouth rinses have been formulated and used for many years, but with as yet little evidence to support their use. One commonly employed is 'Magic mouthwash' consisting of a mixture of viscous lidocaine, benadryl, and aluminium hydroxide. This regimen was evaluated in comparison with standard mouth care with salt and soda rinses and found to have no added benefit in patients receiving stomatotoxic chemotherapy.[48] Although not studied independently, viscous lidocaine has been used with anecdotal success in the control of mucositis pain. Topical application prior to meals or with phonation can decrease pain; however, care must be taken to prevent anaesthesia of airway reflexes with inadvertent administration to the posterior pharynx or trachea. This latter risk remains largely theoretical; however, with a high prevalence of impaired swallowing reflexes and silent aspiration seen in association with cancer treatment alone—78 and 22% in one study[49]—the potential increased risk of aspiration with the use of viscous lidocaine should be borne in mind.

Other

A number of other potentially beneficial therapies have been examined in an attempt either to decrease the extent of mucositis or to manage the accompanying pain. Ketamine has been used successfully in a case report.[50]

The N-methyl-D-aspartate (NMDA) antagonism action of ketamine is thought to be the neurophysiological basis of its analgesic effect in subanaesthetic dose, by reducing 'wind-up' pain and hyperalgesia refractory to standard analgesics. Several reports of its analgesic effect outline the risk of a variety of adverse effects, including a very unpleasant dissociative state.[51–54] Granulocyte–macrophage colony-stimulating factor (GM-CSF) has been used in both the chemotherapy (high dose setting) and radiation-induced mucositis groups to varying effects.[55,56] In preclinical work, GM-CSF stimulates proliferation of keratino-cytes and endothelial cells, both of which are necessary for wound healing. This formed the basis for its study in mucositis. Other growth factors under investi-gation include keratinocyte growth factor, interleukin 11, and transforming growth factor-β.[30] To date, however, none has shown overwhelming success with the possible exception of KGF (palifermin) which has demonstrated a palliative effect in the bone marrow transplant population.[57] Clearly more studies are required to support their routine use.

Osteoradionecrosis (ORN)

ORN is a potential devastating sequela of radical radiotherapy in patients with head and neck cancer. About 5–10% patients are affected to some degree, with approximately 2% of cases being severe. The incidence is greater in dentulous patients and those treated with hyperfractionated schedules. Radiotherapy makes bone hypodynamic and hypovascular, and predisposes to this compli-cation. Presentation can range from asymptomatic bone exposure to severe painful necrosis. Various treatment modalities have been employed, including extended antibiotic regimens, hyperbaric oxygen, ultrasound, and radical resection. No standard evidence-based approach has been widely adopted. ORN is similar in many aspects to the recently described osteochemonecrosis of the mandible being reported with bisphosphonate therapy.[58,59] A 2004 survey conducted by the International Myeloma Foundation of 1203 respond-ents receiving bisphosphonate therapy correlated osteochemonecrosis with underlying dental problems and the use of zoledronic acid.[60] As with ORN, osteochemonecrosis has no one clinically recommended treatment, and indeed the use of resection may worsen the clinical situation.[61]

Sequelae in long-term survivors of head and neck cancer

While treatment-related mucositis is a transient event, other sequelae are more permanent, including dysgeusia (distorted sense of taste), dysphagia, and xerostomia in up to 90% of those treated radically. Each of these has long-term complications, such as weight loss in dysgeusia, aspiration-related infection in dysphagia, and dental caries in xerostomia. Great efforts are underway to limit or prevent these long-term sequlae. These include surgical transposition of the salivary gland, use of intensity-modulated radiotherapy (IMRT),[62,63] and sialogogues including cevilamine[64] and pilocarpine.[65]

Cancer-related pain syndromes

Most often, pain in patients with head and neck cancer is due to a direct consequence of the underlying malignancy. Pain can originate from invasion and ulceration of mucous membranes with consequent stimulation of nociceptors (somatic-type pain) and compression or involvement of peripheral nerves or ganglia (neuropathic-type pain). Direct or distant invasion of bone can also result in pain. There are several cancer-related pain syndromes that are sufficiently common in head and neck patients to warrant detailed description.

Neuralgias

Cranial neuralgias are pain syndromes in the distribution of nerves that carry afferent somatic fibres that supply the head and neck [trigeminal, facial (nervus intermedius), glossopharyngeal, vagus, and cervical dorsal roots C2/3].[66] *Idiopathic neuralgias*—brief stabbing pain not due to cancer—are characterized by a characteristic constellation of symptoms and signs: unilateral electric shock-like stabbing pains that are sudden in onset and brief (seconds in duration); lack of objective neurological deficits; pain restricted to one nerve distribution; absence of pain between attacks; and non-noxious stimuli such as light touch precipitating attacks of pain. While idiopathic neuralgia is decidedly uncommon in head and neck cancer patients, *secondary neuralgia*—neuralgia due to damage caused by cancer or its treatment—is common.

Idiopathic trigeminal neuralgia is thought to be caused by mechanical compression of the nerve usually from a tortuous artery near the brainstem.[67] Painful areas follow divisions of the trigeminal nerve, with the lower face, a combination of V2/3, being the most frequently involved. The trigger is always ipsilateral, involving the anterior face (temperature change, touching, talking, swallowing, chewing), but may be remote from the areas of pain. Consequences can lead to devastating interruptions in quality of life and well-being. Fortunately pharmacotherapy often helps to decrease the intensity and frequency of attacks. Most commonly employed are the antiepileptic agents, particularly carbamazepine (starting dose 100 mg daily increased by 100 every 2 days to 600 or 800 mg daily; uncommonly, higher doses will be needed). Phenytoin and more recently gabapentin have demonstrated therapeutic efficacy. Patients unresponsive to medical management may benefit from nerve blocks or various surgical manipulations including peripheral neurectomy, gangliolysis, tractotomy, or stereotactic radiosurgery. These general treatment approaches can also be used in other cranial neuralgias.

Nervus intermedius (geniculate) neuralgia (the somatic sensory branch of the facial nerve) is characterized by shock-like pains deep in the ear triggered by stimulation of the ear canal or through other benign activities such as swallowing or talking. Diagnosis is clinical or by a diagnostic block of both the glossopharyngeal and trigeminal nerves (direct block of nervus intermedius is impossible). In addition to vascular compression, HSV has been identified as a possible aetiological factor.

Glossopharyngeal neuralgia clinically presents as pain in the pharynx, base of the tongue, or tonsillar fossa sometimes radiating to the ipsilateral ear, angle of the jaw, or neck. Because the proximity of glossopharyngeal-mediated functions to brainstem centres controlling heart rate and blood pressure, autonomic symptoms (such as bradycardia, asystole, or hypotension) may accompany pain attacks, leading to syncope. Triggers involve stimulation of structures innervated by the glossopharyngeal nerve and can be therapeutically confirmed with a local block—keeping in mind that some fibres can travel with the vagus nerve so glossopharyngeal block alone can occasionally give unsatisfactory results.

Superior laryngeal neuralgia—pathology involving the somatic sensory branch of the vagus—results in pain in the pyriform sinus, angle of the jaw, and the side of the thyroid cartilage. Painful attacks are precipitated through laryngeal stimulation (talking, swallowing, or coughing). If other portions of the vagus are involved, symptoms such as hiccoughs, coughing, or autonomic dysfunction may ensue.

Occipital neuralgias, which can result from involvement of the greater or lesser occipital nerves or the second and third cervical roots, are often described as continuous aching and throbbing pain with intermittent shock-like jabs in the occipital region radiating rostrally or laterally. There are no particular triggers, although pressure over the occipital nerves can cause exacerbation.

Other historically described neuralgias including Sluder's and Vidian neuralgia are arguably not distinct phenomena but rather represent unusual presentations of classic neuralgias.

Quite distinct from typical, idiopathic neuralgias are *secondary neuralgias*— neuralgic pains caused by serious underlying pathology such as cancer. In general, patients with a history of head and neck cancer should be assumed to have secondary neuralgia rather than idiopathic neuralgia. Several clinical clues will suggest that there is an underlying cancer: patients often have constant achy pain in between the brief stabbing attacks. Also, the physical examination reveals evidence of sensory disturbance such as numbness, dysaesthesia, or allodynia. The usual mechanism of secondary neuralgias is direct tumour invasion, but occasionally radiation or post-operative nerve damage can be the mechanism. The clinician should be particularly wary of the situation of late onset stabbing neuralgic pain, long after cancer treatment has been completed. Patients who present 3 months or more following definitive treatment of their cancer, with 'out of the blue' onset of neuralgic pain, should be investigated and followed carefully for evidence of recurrent malignancy. However, it may take months for the recurrent cancer to become apparent on physical examination or diagnostic imaging.

Methods of pain control

Successful management of pain relies on correctly identifying the source of pain as this will guide analgesic and oncological interventions, and will inform prognosis. While new innovations are being added to existing treatment options each year, the overall approach remains broadly divided into pharmacological and non-pharmacological strategies.

Ultimately, the ideal management of cancer-induced pain involves identifying the underlying aetiology (i.e. pain due to cancer, due to treatment, or due to neither the cancer nor the treatment) with definitive interventions such as surgery, radiation, and chemotherapy applied as indicated. These same treatment modalities can support symptom control whether or not patients will be likely to be cured of their malignancy.

Drug interventions

The World Health Organization (WHO) analgesia ladder provides a widely accepted framework on which to base initial therapeutic interventions. This approach has resulted in meaningful relief of pain in the large majority of patients.[68] The WHO analgesic ladder describes the use of non-opioids such as acetaminophen (paracetamol) or non-steroidal anti-inflammatory drugs (NSAIDs) for mild pain; and for moderate pain, the addition of 'weak' opioids such as codeine to non-opioids, often in fixed combination preparations. Tramadol is a widely used analgesic, with opioid, serotinergic, and noradrenergic activity, and is generally used at the second step of the ladder. For severe pain or pain that persists despite the application of weak opioids and non-opioids, the third step of the analgesic ladder calls for the use of regularly scheduled administration of a pure opioid agonist such as morphine, in addition to non-opioids or adjuvant analgesics, as indicated.

Table 9.1 Clinical syndromes caused by base of skull metastasis

Syndrome	Structures affected	Pain characteristics	Clinical
Superior orbital fissure syndrome	Superior orbital fissure Cranial nerves III, IV, VI, Ophthalmic branch of V	V-I distribution (eye, supraorbital, lateral nose)	External ophthalmo-plegia (cranial nerves II, IV, VI) Exophthalmos
Retrosphenoidal syndome	Foramen rotundum, foramen ovale, superior orbital fissure, cranial nerves II, III, IV and V	Secondary trigeminal neuralgia	CN III, IV palsy Optic neuropathy Deafness and palatal muscle paralysis
Gasserian ganglion syndrome	Cranial nerve V	VI and VII distribution, dull or lanciating	Tingling in distribution of face Occ CN VI or VII palsy
Pterygopalatine fossa syndrome	Pterygopalatine fossa Maxillary nerve	Neuralgia VII distribu-tion	Maxillary nerve dysaethesias Pterygoid muscle paralysis
Orbintal syndrome	Orbit Cranial nerves III, IV, VI	Dull frontal headache. Secondary trigeminal Neuralgia	CN III, IV, VI palsy Exophthalmos/proptosis Papilloedema
Sphenoid sinus syndrome	Sphenoid sinus CN VI	Bifrontal HA radiation to temples	Nasal congestion CN VI palsy
Cavernous sinus syndrome	Cavernous sinus CN III–VI	Dull aching supra-orbital and frontal V2 distribution	CN III–VI palsy Occ Horner Exophthalmos
Gradenigo—Lannois syndrome	Petrous temporal bone CN V, VI (occ II, IV, VII)	Frontal HA/neuralgia primarily VI	CN V, VI dysfunction
Clivus Jugular foramen	Clivus Narrowing of foramen with dysfunction CN IX–XII and sympathetic nerves	Vertex H/A Pain referred to vertex and ipsilateral arm/shoulder. Occasional glosso-pharyngeal neuralgia	CN VI–XII palsy CN IX–XII palsy Horner's
Occipital condyle syndrome	Occipital condyle CN XII	Unilateral occipital. Aggravated with neck flexion	CN XII palsy
Retroparyngeal syndrome	Retroparotid space SNS CN IX–XII	Retroparotid region Occ glossopharyngeal neuralgia	Horner CN IX, X, XI, XII palsy

(Continued)

Table 9.1 (*Contd.*)

Syndrome	Structures affected	Pain characteristics	Clinical
Cerebellopontine (CPA) syndrome	CN VII–XII Cerebellopontine angle	Occ trigeminal and glossopharyngeal neuralgias	CN VII–XII dysfunction Inc ICP/brainstem compression
Garcin syndrome	Nasopharynx/base of skull All unilateral CN	CN V distribution Nervus intermedius CN IX distribution	Unilateral dysfunction all CN

NSAIDs deserve special mention in the management of pain in patients with head and neck cancer. Because much of the treatment-related pain arises from mucosal inflammation, NSAIDs are widely used. It is believed their effect is through blocking inflammatory mediators of mucositis and consequent nociceptor activation. A trade-off exists, however, with potential benefit being offset by the risk of adverse events in head and neck cancer patients, including bleeding diathesis, dyspepsia, and cardiovascular and renal impairment. These side effects are particularly relevant in the patient receiving cytotoxic or nephrotoxic chemotherapy such as cisplatin.

Opioid analgesics continue to be the cornerstone of managing severe pain. The initial choice of opioid depends on several factors: patient's tolerance to previously prescribed agents, available routes of administration (by mouth; by injection; transdermal; rectal; intravenous; epidural; other), organ function, and intensity and type of pain. While the WHO analgesic ladder has called for morphine as the pure opioid agonist of choice, others may be equally effective. Transdemal fentanyl skin patches have become a popular analgesic in the outpatient setting particularly in patients with pain on swallowing or dysphagia. Limitations include cost and peculiarities related to the transdermal route of opioid administration: a slow onset of action and depot effect. While transdermal opioids can be helpful for chronic baseline pain, an additional strategy needs to be used for breakthrough pain, brief episodes of flairs of pain. Typically, a short-acting oral opioid is used for breakthrough pain. A key issue in the palliative setting is to find an agent that can be effective within a time frame appropriate to the clinical situation. If there is severe pain, either somatic, visceral, or neuropathic, intravenous opioids are the agent of choice because of their speed of onset.

Adjuvant analgesics are frequently used for specific clinical scenarios, such as the use of tricyclics in the management of constant achy neuropathic-type pain.

For brief stabbing pain, sequential trials of carbamazepine, gabapentin, pregabalin, or other anticonvulsants are recommended. Other adjuvant analgesics that are commonly used include: bisphosphonates for bone pain and corticosteroids for the setting of severe pain from metastatic bone disease and pain from bulky tumour recurrence. The use of adjuvant analgesics should be individualized according to the specific clinical scenario. Definitive publications outlining the use of adjuvant analgesics are widely available.[69] Antibiotics can be particularly helpful to reduce head and neck pain if there is bacterial infection.

Drug dependence or drug abuse is an issue frequently feared by patients and their physicians. With adequate pain management, behaviour interpreted as 'drug-seeking' may quickly disappear.[70] Tolerance or the requirement for increasing opioid dosage over time can develop. The escalating opioid dose requirement in a cancer patient is more likely to be secondary to tumour progression than to opioid tolerance.

Interventional pain therapies

Although the majority of cancer-related pain will respond well to the approach outlined by the WHO analgesia ladder, a minority of patients will have *difficult pain problems* and will be candidates for additional pain interventions.[71] These strategies include local delivery of analgesics via an implanted catheter (direct drug delivery), neuroablation, or neurostimulation. With technological advances come the promise of improvements in local treatments, potentially associated with less morbidity compared with equivalent surgical techniques.

Direct drug delivery takes advantage of targeting the source of pain with concentrations of analgesics that would otherwise be systemically intolerable. A common delivery site is the neuraxial via intrathecal or epidural drug administration. Alternatively, regional anaesthesia targeting peripheral nerve structures can be performed. A variety of devices have been employed for these purposes, from simple percutaneous methods to totally implantable devices. There are several limitations to percutaneous devices, including catheter migration or risk of infection, although these routes may be ideal for poor performance status individuals with limited life expectancy. Implantable devices such as epidural or intrathecal catheters require a somewhat more involved surgical procedure and are more suitable for protracted duration of analgesia control. Their use is limited by the effect on diaphragm function.

Neuroablative techniques identify and permanently destroy nerve fibres suspected of mediating the painful stimulus. Indeed this can be used subsequent to local blockade to obviate the need for continuously administered analgesia. Neurolytic procedures typically use surgical, chemical (ethanol, phenol), cryotherapy, or radiofrequency ablation, with the latter receiving much attention due to minimal associated morbidity and improved accuracy.

Finally neurostimulation can be useful in selected patients. The mechanism through which it achieves analgesic effect is postulated to be through stimulation of A-beta fibres which consequently inhibit pain fibres A-delta and C through release of endorphins or enkephalins in the substantial gelatinosa of the dorsolateral funiculus. However, the technique requires surgical placement of a radiofrequency transmitter and electrodes, and may be more suitable for patients with chronic pain syndromes whose life expectancy is sufficiently long to benefit from this intervention.

These techniques have largely supplanted the predominantly surgical approaches employed historically such as multiple rhizotomies, tractotomies, thalamotomies, and psychosurgery (leucotomies, cingulotomies) which were often associated with significant morbidity and mortality.

Summary

Head and neck cancer is commonly associated with pain, right from the time of initial presentation through to treatment, and cure or palliation. Comprehensive patient assessment in order to identify the underlying mechanism is key to constructing an overall management strategy.

References

1 Chaplin, J.M. and Morton, R.P. (1999). A prospective, longitudinal study of pain in head and neck cancer patients. *Head Neck*, 21, 531–537.

2 van Wilgen, C.P., Dijkstra, P.U., van der Laan, B.F,, Plukker, J.T., and Roodenburg, J.L. (2004). Morbidity of the neck after head and neck cancer therapy. *Head Neck*, 26, 785–791.

3 Smit, M., Balm, A.J., Hilgers, F.J., and Tan, I.B. (2001). Pain as sign of recurrent disease in head and neck squamous cell carcinoma. *J Head Neck*, 23, 372–375.

4 Weymuller, E.A., Jr, Yueh, B., Deleyiannis, F.W., *et al.* (2000). Quality of life in head and neck cancer. *Laryngoscope*, 110, 4–7.

5 McDonough, E.M., Varvares, M.A., Dunphy, F.R., Dunleavy, T., Dunphy, C.H., and Boyd, J.H. (1996). Changes in quality-of-life scores in a population of patients treated for squamous cell carcinoma of the head and neck. *Head Neck*, 18, 487–493.

6 Terrell, J.E., Fisher, S.G., and Wolf, G.T. (1998). Long-term quality of life after treatment of laryngeal cancer. The Veterans Affairs Laryngeal Cancer Study Group. *Arch Otolaryngol Head Neck Surg*, 124, 964–971.

7 Bjordal, K., Ohlner-Elmqvist, M., Hammerlid, E., *et al.* (2001). A prospective study of quality of life in head and neck cancer patients. Part II: longitudinal data. *Laryngoscope*, 111, 1440–1452.

8 Fang, F.M., Tsai, W.L., Chien, C.Y., Chiu, H.C., and Wang, C.J. (2004). Health-related quality of life outcome for oral cancer survivors after surgery and postoperative radiotherapy. *Jpn J Clin Oncol*, 34, 641–646.

9 Hagen, N.A., Young, J., and Macdonald, N. (1995). Diffusion of standards of care for care of cancer pain. *J Can Med Assoc*, 152, 1205–1209.

10 Hagen, N.A. (1999). Reproducing a cancer patient's pain on physical examination: bedside provocative maneuvers. *J Pain Symptom Manag*, 18, 406–411.

11 Health Technology Assessment of Positron Emission Tomography (PET) in Oncology— a systematic review. Toronto (ON): Institute for Clinical Evaluative Sciences; 2004. http://www.ices.on.ca/webbuild/site/ices-internet-upload/file_collection/Pet%5Freport% 5FApr%5F2004%5B1%5D%2Epdf.

12 Peterson, D.E. (1992). Oral toxicity of chemotherapeutic agents. *Semin Oncol*, 19, 478–491.

13 Donnelly, J.P., Bell, L.A., Epstein, J.B., Sonis, S.T., and Symonds, R.P. (2003). Antimicrobial therapy to prevent or treat oral mucositis. *Lancet Infect Dis*, 3, 405–412.

14 Redding, S.W. (2005). Cancer therapy-related oral mucositis. *J Dent Educ*, 69, 919–929.

15 Chambers, M.S., Garden, A.S., Kies, M.S., Martin, J.W. (2004). Radiation-induced xerostomia in patients with head and neck cancer: pathogenesis, impact on quality of life, and management. *Head Neck*, 26, 796–807.

16 Meurman, J.H., Pyrhonen, S., Teerenhovi, L., and Lindqvist, C. (1997). Oral sources of septicaemia in patients with malignancies. *J Oral Oncol*, 33, 389–397.

17 Epstein, J.B., Freilich, M.M., and Le, N.D. (1993). Risk factors for oropharyngeal candidiasis in patients who receive radiotherapy for malignant conditions of the head and neck. *Oral Surg Oral Med Oral Pathol*, 76, 169–174.

18 Cooper, J.S., Pajak, T.F., Forastiere, A.A., *et al.* (2004). Postoperative concurrent radiotherapy and chemotherapy for high-risk squamous-cell carcinoma of the head and neck. *N Engl J Med*, 350, 1937–1944.

19 Forastiere, A.A., Metch, B., Schuller, D.E., *et al.* (1992). Randomized comparison of cisplatin plus fluorouracil and carboplatin plus fluorouracil versus methotrexate in advanced squamous-cell carcinoma of the head and neck: a Southwest Oncology Group study. *J Clin Oncol*, 10, 1245–1251.

20 Hughes, W.T., Armstrong, D., Bodey, G.P., *et al.* (2002). 2002 guidelines for the use of antimicrobial agents in neutropenic patients with cancer. *Clin Infect Dis*, 34, 730–751.

21 Rossie, K.M., Taylor, J., Beck, F.M., Hodgson, S.E., Blozis, G.G. (1987). Influence of radiotherapy on oral Candida albicans colonization: a quantitative assessment. *Oral Surg Oral Med Oral Pathol* 64, 698–701.

22 Philpott-Howard, J.N., Wade, J.J., Mufti, G.J., Brammer, K.W., and Ehninger, G. (1993). Randomized comparison of oral fluconazole versus oral polyenes for the prevention of fungal infection in patients at risk of neutropenia. Multicentre Study Group. *J Antimicrob Chemother*, 31, 973–984.

23 Young, G.A., Bosly, A., Gibbs, D.L., and Durrant, S. (1999). A double-blind comparison of fluconazole and nystatin in the prevention of candidiasis in patients with leukemia. Antifungal Prophylaxis Study Group. *Eur J Cancer*, 35, 1208–1213.

24 Epstein, J.B., Gorsky, M., Hancock, P., Peters, N., and Sherlock, C.H. (2002). The prevalence of herpes simplex virus shedding and infection in the oral cavity of seropositive

patients undergoing head and neck radiotherapy. *Oral Surg Oral Med Oral Pathol Oral Radiol Endod*, **94**, 712–716.

25 Nicolatou-Galitis, O., Dardoufas, K., Markoulatos, P., *et al.* (2001). Oral pseudomembranous candidiasis, herpes simplex virus-1 infection, and oral mucositis in head and neck cancer patients receiving radiotherapy and granulocyte–macrophage colony-stimulating factor (GM-CSF) mouthwash. *J Oral Pathol Med* **30**, 471–480.

26 Bubley, G.J., Chapman, B., Chapman, S.K., Crumpacker, C.S., and Schnipper, L.E. (1989). Effect of acyclovir on radiation- and chemotherapy-induced mouth lesions. *Antimicrob Agents Chemother*, **33**, 862–865.

27 Redding, S.W., Luce, E.B., and Boren, M.W. (1990). Oral herpes simplex virus infection in patients receiving head and neck radiation. *Oral Surg Oral Med Oral Pathol*, **69**, 578–580.

28 Redding, S.W. and Montgomery, M.T. (1989). Acyclovir prophylaxis for oral herpes simplex virus infection in patients with bone marrow transplants. *Oral Surg Oral Med Oral Pathol*, **67**, 680–683.

29 Carl, W. and Havens, J. (2000). The cancer patient with severe mucositis. *Curr Rev Pain*, **4**, 197–202.

30 Filicko, J., Lazarus, H.M., and Flomenberg, N. (2003). Mucosal injury in patients undergoing hematopoietic progenitor cell transplantation: new approaches to prophylaxis and treatment. *J Bone Marrow Transplant*, **31**, 1–10.

31 Scully, C., Epstein, J., and Sonis, S. (2003). Oral mucositis: a challenging complication of radiotherapy, chemotherapy, and radiochemotherapy: part 1, pathogenesis and prophylaxis of mucositis. *Head Neck*, **25**, 1057–1070.

32 Scully, C., Epstein, J., and Sonis, S. (2004). Oral mucositis: a challenging complication of radiotherapy, chemotherapy, and radiochemotherapy. Part 2: diagnosis and management of mucositis. *Head Neck*, **26**, 77–84.

33 Capizzi, R.L. (1999). The preclinical basis for broad-spectrum selective cytoprotection of normal tissues from cytotoxic therapies by amifostine. *Semin Oncol*, **26**, 3–21.

34 Brizel, D.M., Wasserman, T.H., Henke, M., *et al.* (2000). Phase III randomized trial of amifostine as a radioprotector in head and neck cancer. *J Clin Oncol*, **18**, 3339–3345.

35 Hodson, D.I., Browman, G.P., Thephamongkhol, K., Oliver, T., Zuraw L, and members of the head and neck disease site group (2004). The role of amifostine as a radioprotectant in the management of patients with squamous cell head and neck cancer. Practice guideline report #5–8. Internet Communication.

36 Mahood, D.J., Dose, A.M., Loprinzi, C.L., *et al.* (1991). Inhibition of fluorouracil-induced stomatitis by oral cryotherapy. *J Clin Oncol*, **9**, 449–452.

37 Okuno, S.H., Foote, R.L., Loprinzi, C.L., *et al.* (1997). A randomized trial of a nonabsorbable antibiotic lozenge given to alleviate radiation-induced mucositis. *Cancer*, **79**, 2193–2199.

38 Symonds, R.P., McIlroy, P., Khorrami, J., *et al.* (1996). The reduction of radiation mucositis by selective decontamination antibiotic pastilles: a placebo-controlled double-blind trial. *Br J Cancer*, **74**, 312–317.

39 Foote, R.L., Loprinzi, C.L., Frank, A.R., *et al.* (1994). Randomized trial of a chlorhexidine mouthwash for alleviation of radiation-induced mucositis. *J Clin Oncol*, **12**, 2630–2633.

40 Epstein, J.B., Silverman, S., Jr, Paggiarino, D.A., *et al.* (2001). Benzydamine HCl for prophylaxis of radiation-induced oral mucositis: results from a multicenter, randomized, double-blind, placebo-controlled clinical trial. *Cancer,* 92, 875–885.

41 Epstein, J.B., Stevenson-Moore, P., Jackson, S., Mohamed, J.H., and Spinelli, J.J. (1989). Prevention of oral mucositis in radiotherapy: a controlled study with benzydamine hydrochloride rinse. *Int J Radiat Oncol Biol Phys,* 16, 1571–1575.

42 Kim, J.H., Chu, F.C., Lakshmi, V., and Houde, R. (1986). Benzydamine HCl, a new agent for the treatment of radiation mucositis of the oropharynx. *Am J Clin Oncol,* 9, 132–134.

43 Bianco, J.A., Appelbaum, F.R., Nemunaitis, J., *et al.* (1991). Phase I–II trial of pentoxifylline for the prevention of transplant-related toxicities following bone marrow transplantation. *Blood* 78, 1205–1211.

44 Attal, M., Huguet, F., Rubie, H., *et al.* (1993). Prevention of regimen-related toxicities after bone marrow transplantation by pentoxifylline: a prospective, randomized trial. *Blood,* 82, 732–736.

45 Lievens, Y., Haustermans, K., Van den, W.D., *et al.* (1998). Does sucralfate reduce the acute side-effects in head and neck cancer treated with radiotherapy? A double-blind randomized trial. *Radiother Oncol,* 47, 149–153.

46 Carter, D.L., Hebert, M.E., Smink, K., Leopold, K.A., Clough, R.L., and Brizel, D.M. (1999). Double blind randomized trial of sucralfate vs. placebo during radical radiotherapy for head and neck cancers. *Head Neck,* 21, 760–766.

47 Smith, T. (2001). Gelclair managing the symptoms of oral mucositis. *Hosp Med,* 62, 623–626.

48 Dodd, M.J., Dibble, S.L., Miaskowski, C., *et al.* (2000). Randomized clinical trial of the effectiveness of 3 commonly used mouthwashes to treat chemotherapy-induced mucositis. *Oral Surg Oral Med Oral Pathol Oral Radiol Endod,* 90, 39–47.

49 Hughes, P.J., Scott, P.M., Kew, J., *et al.* (2000). Dysphagia in treated nasopharyngeal cancer. *Head Neck,* 22, 393–397.

50 Slatkin, N.E. and Rhiner, M. (2003). Topical ketamine in the treatment of mucositis pain. *Pain Med,* 4, 298–303.

51 Fitzgibbon, E.J. and Viola, R. (2005). Parenteral ketamine as an analgesic adjuvant for severe pain: development and retrospective audit of a protocol for a palliative care unit. *J Palliat Med,* 8, 49–57.

52 Elia, N. and Tramer, M.R. (2005). Ketamine and postoperative pain—a quantitative systematic review of randomised trials. *Pain,* 113, 61–70.

53 Bell, R.F., Eccleston, C. and Kalso, E. (2003). Ketamine as adjuvant to opioids for cancer pain. A qualitative systematic review. *J Pain Symptom Manag,* 26, 867–875.

54 Fisher, K., Coderre, T.J., and Hagen, N.A. (2000). Targeting the N-methyl-D-aspartate receptor for chronic pain management. Preclinical animal studies, recent clinical experience and future research directions. *J Pain Symptom Manag,* 20, 358–373.

55 Wagner, W., Alfrink, M., Haus, U., and Matt, J. (1999). Treatment of irradiation-induced mucositis with growth factors (rhGM-CSF) in patients with head and neck cancer. *Anticancer Res,* 19, 799–803.

56 Nemunaitis, J., Rosenfeld, C.S., Ash, R., *et al.* (1995). Phase III randomized, double-blind placebo-controlled trial of rhGM-CSF following allogeneic bone marrow transplantation. *Bone Marrow Transplant,* 15, 949–54.

57 Spielberger, R., Stiff, P., Bensinger, W., Gentile, T., Weisdorf, D., Kewalramani, T., *et al.* (2004). Palifermin for oral mucositis after intensive therapy for hematologic cancers. *N Engl J Med* 351, 2590–8.

58 Marx, R.E. (2003). Pamidronate (Aredia) and zoledronate (Zometa) induced avascular necrosis of the jaws: a growing epidemic. *J Oral Maxillofac Surg*, 61, 1115–1117.

59 Marx, R.E., Sawatari, Y., Fortin, M., and Broumand, V. (2005). Bisphosphonate-induced exposed bone (osteonecrosis/osteopetrosis) of the jaws: risk factors, recognition, prevention, and treatment. *J Oral Maxillofac Surg*, 63, 1567–1575.

60 Durie, B.G., Katz, M., and Crowley, J. (2005). Osteonecrosis of the jaw and bisphosphonates. *N Engl J Med*, 353, 99–102.

61 Ruggiero, S.L., Mehrotra, B., Rosenberg, T.J., and Engroff, S.L. (2004). Osteonecrosis of the jaw associated with the use of bisphosphonates: a review of 63 cases. *J Oral Maxillofac Surg*, 62, 527–534.

62 Kam, M.K., Leung, S.F., Zee, B., *et al.* (2005). Impact of intensity-modulated radiotherapy (IMRT) on salivary gland function in early-stage nasopharygeal carcinoma (NPC) patients: a prospective randomized study. *Proc Am Soc Clin Oncol*, Abstract 5501.

63 Rudat, V., Munter, M., Rades, D., *et al.* (2005). The effect of amifostine or IMRT to preserve the parotid function after radiotherapy of the head and neck region measured by quantitative salivary gland scintigraphy. *Proc Am Soc Clin Oncol*, Abstract 5502.

64 Chambers, M.S., Posner, M.R., Jones, C.U., Weber, R.S., and Vitti, R. (2005). Two phase III clinical studies of Cevimeline for post-radiation xerostomia in patients with head and neck cancer. *Proceedings of the American Society of Clinical Oncology* 23, 500s.

65 Porter, S.R., Scully, C., and Hegarty, A.M. (2004). An update of the etiology and management of xerostomia. *Oral Surg Oral Med Oral Pathol Oral Radiol Endod*, 97, 28–46.

66 Hagen, N.A. and Kauffman, A. (1999). The neuralgias. In Joynt R, Griggs R, eds, *J Baker's Clinical Neurology* on CD-ROM. Philadelphia, Lippincott-Williams & Wilkins.

67 Sens, M.A. and Higer, H.P. (1991). MRI of trigeminal neuralgia: initial clinical results in patients with vascular compression of the trigeminal nerve. *J Neurosurg*, 14, 69–73.

68 Jadad, A.R. and Browman, G.P. (1995). The WHO analgesic ladder for cancer pain management. Stepping up the quality of its evaluation. *J Am Med Assoc* 274, 1870–1873.

69 Lussier, D. and Portenoy, R.K. (2004). Adjuvant analgesics in pain management. In Doyle, D., Calman, K., Hanks, G., and Chernyl, N., eds. *Oxford textbook of palliative medicine*, 3rd edn., pp. 349–378. New York, Oxford University Press.

70 Portenoy, R.K. (1996). Opioid therapy for chronic nonmalignant pain: a review of the critical issues. *J Pain Symptom Manag*, 11, 203–217.

71 Kim, P. S. (2005). Interventional cancer pain therapies. *Semin Oncol* 32, 194–9.

Chapter 10

Psychological issues in advanced or recurrent disease

Maria Frampton and Declan Lyons

Introduction

The diagnosis of cancer carries with it the threat of multiple losses, including loss of bodily parts, loss of bodily functions, loss of personal role, and, especially, loss of life. It is therefore not surprising that severe psychological reactions may be provoked by this group of diseases.

Cancer of the head and neck region may be even more traumatic than other types of cancer, as the disease and treatment thereof can adversely affect highly visible, meaningful, social functions such as speaking, eating, and drinking. Moreover, unlike many other forms of cancer, the disfigurement associated with head and neck cancer cannot easily be hidden from view.

The first part of the chapter will discuss the general aspects, whilst the second part of the chapter will discuss common forms, of psychological/psychiatric disturbance encountered by patients with head and neck cancer.

Epidemiology

Psychological distress is very common in patients with cancer, but formal psychiatric disorders are also common in this group of patients. Derogatis *et al.* used standardized psychiatric interviews and a self-rating symptom checklist (the SCL-90) to determine the psychiatric morbidity in 215 cancer in-patients.[1] Of the patients, 44% were judged to be suffering from a psychiatric illness; of these patients, 68% were categorized as suffering from an 'adjustment disorder' (see below), 13% from a major depression, and 4% from an anxiety disorder. It should be noted that depression, or anxiety, was the predominant symptom in 85% of the patients with an adjustment disorder.

Studies involving head and neck patients have also reported significant levels of psychological distress/psychiatric disorders. In particular, oropharyngeal cancers have been found to be highly associated with depression, with reported prevalence rates ranging from 22 to 57% (and being higher than those of most other types of cancer).[2] However, the tendency of health care professionals to identify with their patients, and to accept depression as 'understandable', may lead to the diagnosis of depression being delayed or missed altogether. For instance, Berard and colleagues, in a study of 456 cancer out-patients, found that only 14% of patients with demonstrable depression had already been identified and treated for the depression.[3]

Other psychiatric disorders that are also common in this group of patients include anxiety disorders, and organic mental disorders (e.g. alcohol with-drawal and other forms of delirium).

Aetiology

Potential predictors of psychological/psychiatric problems include a com-bination of patient-related factors, disease-related factors, and treatment-related factors, together with factors pertaining to the patient's environment.[4] Figure 10.1 demonstrates some of the important factors associated with psychological/psychiatric problems in patients with head and neck cancer.[5]

It is possible to develop a predictive model to identify patients that are particularly likely to experience difficulties. As a result, relevant interventions can be targeted at high risk individuals in the hope of preventing subsequent morbidity. However, in addition to the aforementioned factors, current psy-chological stresses which are not related to the illness also need to be taken into account.

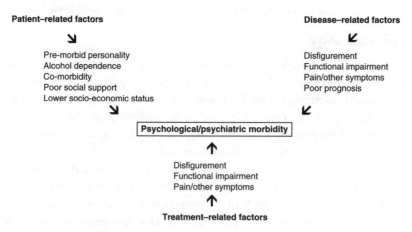

Fig. 10.1 Factors associated with psychological morbidity in patients with head and neck cancer (Frampton[5]).

For example, De Leeuw and colleagues found that certain pre-treatment variables were of predictive value in terms of identifying those head and neck cancer patients who were likely to become depressed in the 3 years following treatment:[6] (1) female gender; (2) advanced tumour stage; (3) presence of tumour-related symptoms; (4) presence of depressive symptoms; (5) lack of openness to discussing cancer within the family; (6) lack of emotional support; and (7); small size of informal social network.

Patient-related factors

Studies have found that while older people may encounter more practical limitations as a result of their illness and treatment, they may experience less existential distress (and less depression).[7]

Certain personality types have been associated with maladaptive responses.[8] For example, people with a so-called narcissistic personality organization (i.e. individuals who pride themselves in possessing unusual attractiveness, and whose self-esteem largely rests on such characteristics) may be at risk of severe depression if they develop a facial cancer, or a treatment-related disfigurement.

Disease-related factors

The risk of recurrence of orofacial cancer is relatively high in comparison with other malignancies, and fear of recurrence, and uncertainty regarding prognosis, are strongly associated with psychological morbidity.[9]

Treatment-related factors

In terms of discriminating between the effects of different treatments in causing psychological distress in patients, many studies have methodological limitations such as failure to take pre-existing personality traits, coping styles, or psychiatric morbidity into account, as well as combining small numbers of patients with different forms and stages of cancer. Nevertheless, studies have shown that psychological outcome is better in those patients treated by non-operative methods, particularly in those patients presenting with advanced disease.[10]

In addition, the extent of visible surgical resection is important in terms of the psychosocial impact of treatment. Dhillon et al. examined the impact of laryngectomy and the 'commando procedure' in an uncontrolled study of patients with cancer of the larynx.[11] (The commando procedure involves excision of the tumour, excision of half the lower jaw bone, and a radical neck dissection.) The study indicated that the commando procedure led to more problems related to eating and drinking, and also to severe dribbling.

Furthermore, the more visible nature of the problems experienced by the commando patients resulted in more of these patients becoming social recluses (43% compared with 11%), and experiencing frequent or constant episodes of depression (21% compared with 14%).

It is important that patients receive adequate/honest pre-treatment counselling to prepare them for the physical and psychological changes which will occur as a result of the treatment.[12]

General aspects of management

Case finding

Case finding is the cornerstone of management. As discussed above, one of the major factors for the delay in diagnosing patients as having a formal psychiatric disorder is the tendency for health care professionals to accept reactions such as anxiety and low mood as being understandable in the circumstances.

Other clinician factors that mitigate against the early detection of psychiatric illness include fears of asking patients about their concerns, fears about their own lack of counselling skills (i.e. that they will not be able to deal with problems that emerge), and fears about being unsupported if they choose to explore any such concerns.[13]

The use of validated screening instruments should help to overcome the former issue (see below), whilst the inclusion of relevant health care professionals in the multidisciplinary head and neck team should help to overcome the latter issues (e.g. liaison psychiatrists, clinical psychologists).

Multidisciplinary working

Ideally, the multidisciplinary head and neck team should include health care professionals with the necessary skills/experience to deal with the psychological/psychiatric problems encountered in this group of patients (e.g. liaison psychiatrists, clinical psychologists, counsellors, and social workers).

Nevertheless, health care professionals who have a long-standing relationship with the patient are sometimes in a better position to provide psychological support than a newly arrived liaison psychiatrist or clinical psychologist. This is particularly true during the latter phases of the illness. Indeed, even the most inexperienced professional in terms of counselling skills can offer sympathy and companionship, and consequently all the support that is needed, during this trying time for the patient.

In the terminal phase, dealing with emotions may be challenging, not least because the patient may openly express a loss of confidence in the treating team upon re-emergence of the cancer. However, it is imperative that such patients continue to be supported by the head and neck cancer team. Indeed, patients and their families often obtain remarkable psychological benefit from the simple reassurance of the treating team's availability, and their ongoing commitment to addressing the patient's symptoms/problems.[14]

Psychotherapy

Social supports may buffer some of the burdens and strains associated with the condition, but formal psychotherapy, both cognitive and behavioural, is helpful in the less unwell population of terminally ill patients.[15] Support groups may also provide invaluable informal reassurance, and the team should be encouraging of their patient's participation in such groups.

Adjuvant psychological therapy (APT) is a problem-focused, cognitive–behavioural treatment that was demonstrated to be more effective than supportive counselling in a group of patients with various types and stages of cancer, who met the criteria for an abnormal adjustment reaction.[16] APT produced a significantly greater change in fighting spirit, ability to cope with the cancer, anxiety, and other self-defined problems.

When such formal therapies are not available, or the patient is too debilitated for such therapies, then the head and neck team can still provide important support through showing interest and concern, facilitating the expression of feelings and fears, offering encouragement, and most importantly through the assurance of continuity in care to both the patient and their support network.

A further strategy that can be useful in the terminal phase is to 'remove death from the psychological present'.[17] This stance involves encouraging the patient to complete unfinished business, and so restoring them from a position of passivity (waiting to die) to one of activity (continuing to live).[18]

Anxiety

Clinical features

Anxiety is a particularly common problem during critical moments in the course of cancer treatment, for example while waiting to hear about a possible recurrence of the cancer. Such anxiety may disrupt a patient's ability to function normally, interfere with interpersonal relationships, and even impact on their ability to understand or comply with cancer treatment.

Moreover, in a proportion of patients with facial disfigurement, overwhelming anxiety in relation to concerns about body image will set up panic and avoidance, leading to the development of a generalized or phobic anxiety disorder.

In a recent study, 22% of patients were diagnosed with post-traumatic stress disorder 6 months after the initial diagnosis of head and neck cancer. Patients reported troublesome symptoms, including emotional hyperarousal, persistent reliving of the traumatic experience (e.g. telling of the diagnosis, period on the ICU), and subsequent avoidance of the traumatic stimuli.[19]

Assessment

See section on depression.

Management

Optimal treatment of anxiety without an obvious organic contribution incorporates both a benzodiazepine, and relaxation exercises or other behavioural interventions.[20] The benzodiazepines most commonly used for treatment of anxiety in the oncology setting are alprazolam, clonazepam, and lorazepam. Alprazolam can be used sublingually in patients who have difficulty swallowing.

Non-benzodiazepine anxiolytics may be indicated if there are concerns regarding respiratory depression, or when an underlying organic aetiology is suspected. Both typical and atypical antipsychotic agents are potentially suitable treatments in these situations.

Patients in acute pain or respiratory distress often appear intensely anxious, but generally respond to adequate analgesia or oxygen with or without tailored doses of morphine, respectively. Nevertheless, benzodiazepines may have a role in the management of certain types of acute pain (i.e. muscle spasm), and respiratory distress (i.e. 'panic attacks').

Depression

Many patients experience a low mood, but do not develop a depressive illness, in response to stressors such as receiving bad news. This type of emotional reaction is called an 'adjustment disorder', since there is a clear relationship to a stressor, and the reaction is limited in its duration. In addition, the symptoms of an adjustment disorder often fluctuate, and patients can be distracted, albeit temporarily, from their distress.[21]

Clinical features

The DSM-IV criteria for a major depressive episode are the presence of five (or more) of the following symptoms, including either depressed mood or loss of interest or pleasure in activities, for most of the time in the preceding 2 weeks:[22] (1) depressed mood; (2) loss of interest or pleasure in activities;

(3) weight loss or gain (change of >5% of body weight in 1 month); (4) sleep disorder (insomnia or hypersomnia); (5) fatigue or loss of energy; (6) feelings of worthlessness, or excessive or inappropriate guilt; (7) diminished ability to concentrate or make decisions; and (8) recurrent thoughts of death or suicidal ideation, plan, or attempt.

In general, the symptoms of most use in diagnosing depression in the severely physically ill are those which relate to mood, thought content, and suicidal feelings. Indeed, Endicott proposed an alternative set of criteria for use in cancer patients, which involved replacing the aforementioned somatic symptoms.[23] Thus, Endicott replaced change in weight with observation of a fearful or depressed appearance; sleep disturbance with social withdrawal or decreased talkativeness; loss of energy with brooding, self-pity, or pessimism; and poor concentration with a mood non-reactive to environmental events.

Assessment

A number of screening instruments have been assessed for their utility in terms of detecting anxiety and depression in cancer patients. The General Health Questionnaire 28 (GHQ 28), the Hospital Anxiety and Depression Scale (HADS), and the Rotterdam Symptom Checklist (RSCL) have been most frequently compared.[5] These screening instruments possess a high degree of sensitivity, i.e. one can say with a high degree of confidence that patients with a negative test are highly unlikely to have, for example, depression. However, the screening instruments may have differential sensitivity depending on whether the patient has active disease or not, and/or whether they are currently undergoing treatment or not. Self-reporting instruments such as the GHQ, or the Beck's Depression Inventory, are gaining more favour, as they are brief, convenient, and easily completed, even by severely ill patients.[24] Such questionnaires can be used in hospital wards and out-patient clinics to identify patients likely to have a mental illness, and so require further assessment and treatment.

Management

Depression in cancer patients is optimally managed with a combination of supportive psychotherapy, cognitive–behavioural techniques, and antidepressant medications.[25] However, it is important also to address any reversible factors contributing to the depression (e.g. pain, other symptoms). Indeed, adequate symptom control is one of the cornerstones in the treatment of depression at the end of life.

As discussed above, some patients that are low in mood may be experiencing an adjustment disorder, rather than a depressive illness. Thus, in patients who have experienced a recent stressor such as receiving bad news, it may be appropriate to delay treatment and review the patient in 2–3 weeks. However, in patients with insufficient time to 'wait and see', an early trial of an antidepressant may be warranted. Other factors such as a past history of depression, a family history of mood disorders, and a previous response to treatment may also prompt the decision to offer early treatment.

When treating a patient with a major depressive disorder, it may be more appropriate to delay commencing formal psychotherapy until the antidepressant treatment has started to work, as severely depressed people may be unable to reflect objectively on their situation, and any psychological intervention may increase introspection and negative rumination, and hence worsen the depressive symptoms.[26]

Antidepressant drugs are effective in 65–75% of patients, and their efficacy has been well established in cancer patients.[27] The main classes of antidepressants in current use are the tricyclic antidepressants (TCAs), the selective serotonin re-uptake inhibitors (SSRIs), the serotonin and noradrenaline re-uptake inhibitors (SNRIs), and the noradrenergic and specific serotonergic antidepressants (NaSSAs).[28] Other drugs/groups of drugs, such as lithium and the monoamine oxidase inhibitors (MAOIs), are generally reserved for special circumstances and refractory cases.

There are few controlled trials of antidepressant drug therapies in patients with cancer. Thus, general principles have to be followed when prescribing for this group of patients. The choice of agent depends on the patient's presenting symptom profile, the patient's likely tolerability of the drug, and potential drug interactions. It is also important to consider the secondary effects of the agent, since these may provide additional positive worth. For instance, in the case of an agitated patient, who has difficulty sleeping, a sedating antidepressant would be particularly useful (e.g. amitriptyline, mirtazepine).[29]

In the terminal phase, another important factor affecting the choice of agent is the speed of onset of action. Conventional antidepressants take 2–4 weeks to achieve an effect, which may be too long for some patients. In such cases, it may be worth considering the use of a psychostimulant drug (e.g. methylphenidate dexamphetamine).[30] Psychostimulants can have a rapid onset of action, with some patients improving within a few doses of the drug. Psychostimulants can also be used as a 'stop gap', whilst waiting for a conventional antidepressants to achieve an effect.

Patients who are unable to swallow tablets may be able to take an antidepressant in elixir form (e.g. amitriptyline, paroxetine). Parenteral administration of tricyclic antidepressants can be considered for the cancer patient unable to tolerate oral administration, but close monitoring of cardiac conduction by electrocardiograph (ECG) is recommended when these drugs are used intravenously. Clinicians unaccustomed to initiating psychotropic medication are advised to consult a relevant formulary (e.g. *British National Formulary*[28]) or prescribing guide (e.g. *The Maudsley 2005–2006 Prescribing Guidelines*[31]]).

Suicidal ideation

Suicidal thoughts are not unusual in patients with life-threatening diagnoses, but a pervasive desire for death should be regarded as abnormal. The risk of suicide increases with advancing illness, and an old survey by Farberow and colleagues found that 86% of suicides occurred in the terminal phase of a cancer.[32]

If a patient reports suicidal ideation, then the initial priority is to sit down with them and explore the meaning of the suicidal thoughts, as well as evaluate the risk of suicide. Suicide vulnerability factors can be used as a guide in evaluating the risk of suicide (see Box 10.1).[20] Allowing the patient to discuss suicidal thoughts often decreases the risk of suicide, and there is absolutely no evidence that asking about suicidal thoughts 'puts the idea into their head'.

The goal of intervention is to deal with the issues that are contributing to the suicidal ideation. Management of depression can dramatically improve the quality of life of the patient, reduce feelings of hopelessness, and, in turn, reduce the desire for death and also the risk of suicide.[33] Aggressive treatment of pain and other symptoms can also help turn the tide for individual patients.

Box 10.1. **Cancer suicide vulnerability factors (Breitbart[13])**

Pain, suffering aspects

Advanced illness; poor prognosis

Depression; hopelessness

Delirium; disinhibition

Control; helplessness

Pre-existing psychopathology

Suicide history; family history

Inadequate social support

If the patient is actively suicidal, then a 24 h companion or nurse may be appropriate to monitor the suicidal risk, and also to provide reassurance for the patient.

Delirium

Delirium and other organic mental disorders occur in 15–20% of hospitalized cancer patients, are the second most common group of psychiatric diagnoses ascribed to cancer patients, and are particularly common in patients with advanced disease.[34]

Delirium may be precipitated by the direct effects of the cancer on the central nervous system (CNS), or by indirect CNS effects of the disease or treatments, including medication effects, concomitant infection, organ failure, or vascular complications. Opioid analgesics (e.g. morphine sulfate), corticosteroids, and some chemotherapeutic agents have all been reported to cause confusional states, especially in the elderly and in terminally ill cancer patients.[35]

Clinical features

Delirium has been described as an aetiologically non-specific, global, cerebral dysfunction characterized by concurrent disturbances in any number of different functions, including level of consciousness, attention, thinking, perception, emotion, memory, psychomotor behaviour, and the sleep–wake cycle.[20] Thus the clinical features of delirium can include poor cooperation with care, poor concentration, confusion, apathy, anxiety, depression, withdrawal, anger, and psychosis.

Heavy alcohol consumption is an important pre-morbid risk factor for head and neck cancer, and alcohol misuse may also have become a maladaptive coping mechanism for the ongoing problems associated with the cancer. Hence, alcohol withdrawal is a significant cause of delirium in this group of patients ('delirium tremens'). The signs and symptoms of alcohol withdrawal are typical of general delirium, and include the development of clouding of consciousness, disorientation, psychomotor agitation, and perceptual disturbances in any modality, but especially visual hallucinations. In addition, alcohol withdrawal can also be associated with seizures. It should be noted that the onset of these clinical features may be delayed by up to a week after the last consumption of alcohol.[36]

Assessment

Mental test batteries, such as the Mini-Mental State Examination, are sensitive to the presence of delirium.[18] Assessment may be affected by compromised communication. However, even tracheostomized patients should be able to nod yes or no, to write, and to follow relevant commands, and thus be able to complete such an assessment satisfactorily.

Distinguishing delirium from dementia may be difficult as many clinical features such as disorientation, impaired memory, and impaired judgement are shared. However, dementia is typically more insidious in onset and appears in individuals with little or no clouding of consciousness. Delirium can occasionally be superimposed on an underlying dementia, particularly in older patients or patients with a paraneoplastic syndrome.

Management

Delirium is generally conceptualized as being a reversible process. Simple investigations may include biochemical screening, and appropriate investigations to exclude infection. In addition, a simple medication review may be extremely informative. If a reversible cause is identified, then this should be appropriately managed.

The treatment of delirium also includes maintenance of the patient's safety, and symptomatic therapy. Measures to help reduce disorientation and anxiety include explanation, reassurance, and frequent reorientation to their environment by ensuring a familiar and structured routine. The presence of a 'familiar face' may also be very helpful (e.g. family member, close friend).

Neuroleptic and other sedative medications are often necessary to treat the agitation and behavioural problems that accompany delirium. Haloperidol, a high potency neuroleptic, used in small doses, is the preferred drug for treatment of delirium in the cancer patient due to its low incidence of anticholinergic and cardiovascular effects. The usual starting dose is 0.5 mg once or twice daily, with titration according to symptomatology, to the usual level of 3–5 mg per day. Newer antipsychotic drugs such as risperidone and olanzepine are being increasingly utilized, owing to their favourable side effect profiles, i.e. a lesser propensity to cause extrapyramidal symptoms.

Concomitant benzodiazepine medication can be helpful in the treatment of agitation associated with delirium, but only low doses of short-acting agents such as lorazepam are recommended, since these agents have a tendency to accumulate, and may possibly worsen the confusion.

Key points

• Psychological disorders are common amongst head and neck cancer patients, and should not be regarded as 'understandable' and thus not worthy of treatment.

- Common disorders include anxiety and depression, but also organically based disorders such as delirium.

- Screening instruments in the form of questionnaires and rating scales are being increasingly employed to detect anxiety and depression in the cancer population.

- The expertise of Liaison Psychiatry and specialist mental health professionals may be needed, but the original treating surgical or oncological team should continue to remain engaged with the terminally ill patient to offer ongoing psychological support.

- Judicious psychopharmacological interventions, combined with psychological therapies, can achieve significant quality of life improvements even in terminally ill patients.

References

1 Derogatis, L.R., Morrow, G.R., Fetting, J., et al. (1983). The prevalence of psychiatric disorders among cancer patients. *J Am Med Assoc*, **249**, 751–757.

2 Massie, M.J. (2004). Prevalence of depression in patients with cancer. *J Natl Cancer Inst Monogr*, **32**, 57–71.

3 Berard, R.M., Boermeester, F., and Viljoen, G. (1998). Depressive disorders in an out-patient oncology setting: prevalence, assessment, and management. *Psychooncology*, **7**, 112–120.

4 Harrison, J., and Maguire, P. (1994). Predictors of psychiatric morbidity in cancer patients. *Br J Psychiatry*, **165**, 593–598.

5 Frampton, M. (2001). Psychological distress in patients with head and neck cancer: review. *Br J Oral Maxillofac Surg*, **39**, 67–70.

6 De Leeuw, J.R., de Graeff, A., Ros, W.J., Blijham, G.H., Hordijk, G.J., and Winnubst, J.A. (2001). Prediction of depression 6 months to 3 years after treatment of head and neck cancer. *Head Neck*, **23**, 892–898.

7 Hutton, J.M., and Williams, M. (2001). An investigation of psychological distress in patients who have been treated for head and neck cancer. *Br J Oral and Maxillofac Surg*, **39**, 333–339.

8 Turns, D., and Sands, R.G. (1978). Psychological problems of patients with head and neck cancer. *J Prosthet Dent*, **39**, 68–73.

9 Humphris, G.M., Rogers, S., McNally, D., Lee-Jones, C., Brown, J., and Vaughan, D. (2003). Fear of recurrence and possible cases of anxiety and depression in orofacial cancer patients. *Int J Oral Maxillofac Surg*, **32**, 486–491.

10 McDonough, E.M., Boyd, J.H., Varvares, M.A., and Maves, M.D. (1996). Relationship between psychological status and compliance in a sample of patients treated for cancer of the head and neck. *Head Neck*, **18**, 269–276.

11 Dhillon, R.S., Palmer, B.V., Pittam, M.R., and Shaw, H.J. (1982). Rehabilitation after major head and neck surgery—the patients' view. *Clin Otolaryngol Allied Sci*, **7**, 319–324.

12 Burgess, L. (1994). Facing the reality of head and neck cancer. *Nurs Stand*, **8**, 30–34.

13 Maguire, P. (1997). Depression and cancer. In **Robertson, M.M., and Katona, C.L.**, eds. *Depression and physical illness. Perspectives in psychiatry*, Vol. 6, pp. 429–439. Chichester, UK, John Wiley & Sons Ltd,.

14 Swire, N., and George, R.J. (1997). Depression in palliative care. In **Robertson, M.M., and Katona, C.L.**, eds. *Depression and physical illness. Perspectives in psychiatry*, Vol. 6, pp. 443–464. Chichester, UK, John Wiley& Sons Ltd.

15 Meyer, T.J., and Mark, M.M. (1995). Effects of psychosocial interventions with adult cancer patients: a meta-analysis of randomized experiments. *Health Psychol*, **14**, 101–108.

16 Moorey, S., Greer, S., Bliss, J., and Law, M. (1998). A comparison of adjuvant psychological therapy and supportive counselling in patients with cancer. *Psychooncology*, **7**, 218–228.

17 Eissler, K.R. (1955). *The psychiatrist and the dying patient*. New York, International Universities Press.

18 Shapiro, P.A., and Kornfeld, D.S. (1987). Psychiatric aspects of head and neck cancer surgery. *Psychiatr Clin North Am*, **10**, 87–100.

19 Kangas, M., Henry, J.L., and Bryant, R.A. (2005). The relationship between acute stress disorder and posttraumatic stress disorder following cancer. *J Consult Clin Psychol*, **73**, 360–364.

20 Breitbart, W. (1994). Psycho-oncology: depression, anxiety, delirium. *Semin Oncol*, **21**, 754–769.

21 Maguire, P., Faulkner, A., and Regnard, C. (1993). Handling the withdrawn patient— a flow diagram. *Palliat Med*, **7**, 333–338.

22 **American Psychiatric Association** (1994). *The diagnostic and statistical manual of mental disorders*, 4th edn. APA, Washington, DC.

23 Endicott, J. (1984). Measurement of depression in patients with cancer. *Cancer*, **53** (10 Suppl), 2243–2249.

24 Razavi, D., Delvaux, N., Bredart, A., *et al.* (1992). Screening for psychiatric disorders in a lymphoma out-patient population. *Eur J Cancer*, **28A**, 1869–1872.

25 Massie, M.J., and Holland, J.C. (1990). Depression and the cancer patient. *J Clin Psychiatry*, **51** (Suppl), 12–17.

26 Beck, A.T., Rush, A.J., Shaw, B.F., and Emery, G. (1979). *Cognitive therapy of depression*. New York, Guilford Press.

27 Costa, D., Mogos, I., and Toma, T. (1985). Efficacy and safety of mianserin in the treatment of depression of women with cancer. *Acta Psychiatr Scand Suppl*, **320**, 85–92.

28 **Anonymous** (2005). *British national formulary* 50. London, BMJ Publishing Group Ltd and Royal Pharmaceutical Society of Great Britain.

29 Roth, A., Massie, M.J., and Redd, W.H. (2000). Consultation—liaison psychiatry. In **Jacobson, J.J., and Jacobson, A.M.**, eds. *Psychiatric secrets*, 2nd edn., pp. 412–425. Philadelphia, Hanley & Belfus Inc.

30 Breitbart, W., Chochinov, H.M., and Passik, S.D. (2004). Psychiatric symptoms in palliative medicine. In **Doyle, D., Hanks, G., Cherny, N., and Calman K,** eds. *Oxford textbook of palliative medicine*, 3rd edn., pp. 746–771. Oxford, Oxford University Press.

31 Taylor, D., Paton, C., and Kerwin, R. (2005). *The Maudsley 2005–2006 prescribing guidelines*, 8th edn. London, Taylor & Francis.

32 Farberow, N.L., Schneidman, E.S., and Leonard, C.V. (1963). Suicide among general medical and surgical hospital patients with malignant neoplasms. *Medical Bulletin* 9. Washington, DC, US Veterans Administration.

33 Storm, H.H., Christensen, N., and Jensen, O.M. (1992). Suicides among Danish patients with cancer: 1971 to 1986. *Cancer*, **69**, 1507–1512.

34 Bruera, E., Miller, L., and McCalion, S. (1990). Cognitive failure in patients with terminal cancer: a prospective longitudinal study. *Psychosoc Aspects Cancer*, **9**, 308–310.

35 Massie, M.J., Holland, J., and Glass, E. (1983). Delirium in terminally ill cancer patients. *Am J Psychiatry*, **140**, 1048–1050.

36 Semple, D., Smyth, R., Burns, J., Darjee, R., and McIntosh, A. (2005). *Oxford handbook of psychiatry*. Oxford, Oxford University Press.

Chapter 11

The last few days of life

Emma Thompson and Andrew Davies

Introduction

Head and neck cancer patients often present with locally advanced disease, but rarely with distant metastatic disease. Nevertheless, and in spite of all of the developments in oncological practice, the prognosis remains relatively poor in this group of patients (overall 5-year survival ~40%).[1] The poor prognosis is related both to progression of the malignant disease and also to development/progression of associated diseases (e.g. lung cancer, ischaemic heart disease).[2]

Head and neck cancer patients present particular challenges to health care professionals as a result of a variety of disease-related factors (tumour site), treatment-related factors (morbidity), and patient-related factors (co-morbidity).[3] Challenges occur at all stages of the disease, including the terminal phase. However, many of the latter challenges are generic to all cancer patients, and not specific to head and neck cancer patients.

The aim of this chapter is to review the literature on the terminal phase of head and neck cancer patients, and to provide some practical advice about the management of common problems that may be encountered during this period. Readers are advised to consult an appropriate textbook of palliative care for advice about the management of other relevant problems.[4,5]

The concept of a 'good death'

Most individuals want to experience a 'good death', and have a clear idea about what constitutes such a death. Nevertheless, the concept of a good death varies between individuals, and is influenced by such factors as personal circumstances, religion, and culture.[6] Importantly, there are discrepancies between what health care professionals and non-health care professionals (i.e. patients, patients' families, the general population, and other professionals) consider to be a good death.[7–10]

Steinhauser et al. identified factors important for a good death from four different groups of people: (1) seriously ill patients; (2) recently bereaved families; (3) doctors; and (4) other professionals (e.g. nurses, social workers).[9] The factors that were common to all the groups were:

* adequate pain/symptom control
* clear decisions about management
* being treated as a 'whole person'
* making preparations for death
* achieving a sense of completion.

A number of other factors were highlighted by the group of seriously ill patients, including being mentally alert, not being a burden, planning funeral arrangements and coming to peace with God.

The specialty of palliative care developed as a result of deficiencies in the care of dying patients. The model of care that was adopted was one of holistic care, since it was apparent that the experience of patients was dependent on the interaction of physical, psychological, social, and spiritual factors (see Fig. 11.1). Indeed, different factors take precedence in different patients. The general consensus is that specialist palliative care has improved the end-of-life care of cancer patients, and there is increasing research evidence to back up this impression.[11] However, a significant proportion of cancer patients do not receive specialist palliative care at the end of life.

In an attempt to address the latter issue, a number of end-of-life pathways have been developed/introduced in both the primary care setting (e.g. Macmillan Gold Standards Framework[12]) and the secondary care setting (e.g. Liverpool Integrated Care Pathway[13]). Currently, however, there is little research into the effectiveness of such pathways.[14] In addition, various organizations have produced recommendations/guidelines on end-of-life care. For example, Box. 11.1 demonstrates the principles of high quality end-of-life care

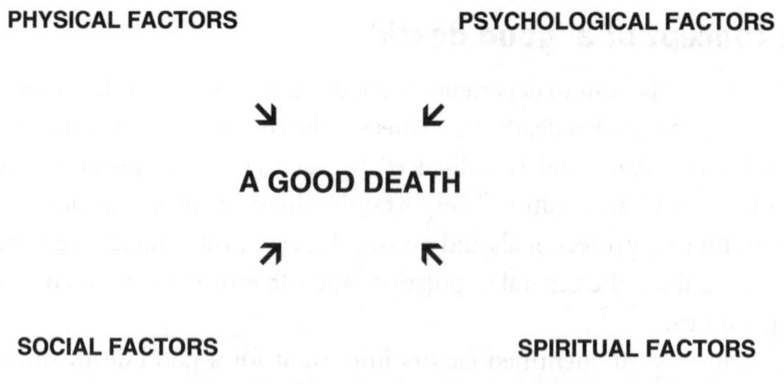

PHYSICAL FACTORS   PSYCHOLOGICAL FACTORS

↘   ↙

A GOOD DEATH

↗   ↖

SOCIAL FACTORS   SPIRITUAL FACTORS

Fig. 11.1 Factors influencing a 'good death'.

as described by the American Medical Association (and endorsed by the American Society of Clinical Oncology).[15]

The reality of death

Many head and neck patients are hospitalized during the last few months of life, and many remain hospitalized during the terminal phase (see below). For example, a study from the UK reported that 53% of patients were hospitalized during the last month of life: the reasons for admission included bleeding episodes (17%), pain problems (9%), breathing difficulties (9%), swallowing difficulties (9%), inability to cope (6%), and a fracture (3%).[16]

In most cases, the terminal phase is relatively straightforward in patients with head and neck cancer.[17] Thus, it is feasible to consider the option of a home death, particularly as the literature suggests that most cancer patients would prefer to die at home. However, it appears that most head and neck cancer patients die in hospital, rather than at home or in other care settings.[16,18,19]

For example, a study from the UK reported that 62% of patients died in a hospital, 19% died in a hospice, 16% died at home, and 3% died in a nursing

---

Box 11.1. American Medical Association Institute for Ethics' elements of quality end of life care.[15]

- The opportunity to discuss and plan end-of-life care.

- Trustworthy assurance that physical and mental suffering will be carefully attended to and comfort measures intently secured.

- Trustworthy assurance that preferences for withholding or withdrawing life-sustaining intervention will be honoured.

- Trustworthy assurance that there will be no abandonment by the physician.

- Trustworthy assurance that dignity will be a priority.

- Trustworthy assurance that burden to family and others will be minimized.

- Attention to the personal goals of the dying process.

- Trustworthy assurance that caregivers will assist the bereaved through the early stages of mourning and adjustment.

home.[16] There are numerous explanations, but minimal information, for the high rate of hospital deaths (and the low rate of home deaths).[20] Nevertheless, a study from Israel reported that patients that died at home were younger and had better symptom control (pain control) than patients that died in a hospital.[21]

In most instances, head and neck cancer patients die as a result of gradual deterioration in their condition.[17,18] Furthermore, as discussed above, the majority of patients have a relatively uneventful terminal phase (i.e. from the health professional view point).[17]Nevertheless, in some instances, head and neck cancer patients die as a result of an acute complication of their disease (e.g. airway obstruction, haemorrhage), or an acute event not directly related to the disease (e.g. myocardial infarction, pulmonary embolism). Table 11.1 demonstrates the reported cause of death amongst a cohort of head and neck cancer patients admitted to a hospice in the UK.[17]

Management—general principles

The problems encountered in the terminal phase are similar to those experienced in other phases of the disease, with the major exceptions of terminal agitation and excess respiratory secretions (so-called 'death rattle). The management of problems needs to be tailored to the change in circumstances, although sometimes 'active' treatment is the most effective form of palliation. For example, it may be appropriate to treat patients with bronchopneumonia with antibiotics in order to improve their symptoms (e.g. cough, dyspnoea), as opposed to trying to prolong their life. The management of terminal agitation and excess respiratory secretions is briefly summarized in Table 11.2.

Table 11.1 Causes of death in head and neck patients receiving palliative care[17]

Cause of death	Number of patients ($n = 36$)
Progressive disease*	17 (47%)
Bronchopneumonia	9 (25%)
Massive haemorrhage	3 (8%)
Airway obstruction	2 (6%)
Myocardial infarction	2 (6%)
Cardiac failure	2 (6%)
Other	1 (2%)

*Condition gradually deteriorated.

Table 11.2 Management of common symptoms in the terminal phase

Symptom	Management options	Comments
Terminal agitation	Treatment of the underlying cause	In certain circumstances it is possible to identify a reversible/treatable cause of the agitation.
	Non-pharmacological interventions 'Environmental interventions'	Patients should be cared for in a quiet, well-illuminated room, which contains objects familiar to the patient (e.g. photographs), and objects that can help to orientate the patient (e.g. clock). In addition, patients are often reassured by the presence of non-professional carers.
	Pharmacological interventions Antipsychotic agents (e.g. haloperidol, levomepromazine) Sedative agents (e.g. midazolam, propofol)	Antipsychotic agents are considered to be the treatment of choice for terminal agitation. Benzodiazepines (e.g. midazolam) are useful in cases associated with anxiety, whilst other sedative drugs (e.g. propofol) are useful in refractory cases.
Excess respiratory secretions ('death rattle')	Non-pharmacological interventions Reassurance (of carers) Repositioning Suctioning	Carers should be informed that although the noise is distressing for them, the excess secretions are invariably not distressing for the patient. Repositioning may be effective and, if there is pooling of secretions in the oropharynx, suctioning may be appropriate/effective.
	Pharmacological interventions Anticholinergic agents (e.g. glycopyrronium bromide, hyoscine hydrobromide)	Anticholinergic drugs are only effective in ~50% of cases. Glycopyrronium bromide is a quaternary amide, and so less likely to cross the blood–brain barrier, and so less likely to cause agitation (cf. hyoscine hydrobromide).

The multidisciplinary approach is as valid in the terminal phase of the illness as in the earlier phases of the illness. Thus, whilst palliative care professionals are experienced in dealing with problems relating to symptom control, they are often less experienced in dealing with problems relating to tracheostomy tubes, or enteral feeding tubes. In addition, the transition from active treatment to palliative care may be made easier by the ongoing support of familiar health care professionals (e.g. head and neck oncology nurse).

Oral administration of medication may become increasingly more difficult during the terminal phase. In some cases, medication can be given via an established enteral feeding tube. The decision to use this route is dependent on a number of factors, including the availability of a suitable formulation of the drug, the compatibility of the drug and the enteral feed, and various practical issues (the position of the feeding tube, the size of the feeding tube).[22] However, in many cases, medication needs to be given via a parenteral route.

The subcutaneous route is the most commonly used parenteral route in palliative care.[22] A subcutaneous cannula can be inserted, which allows repeated administration of drugs, or administration of continuous infusions of drugs. Numerous drugs can be given subcutaneously, although in most cases they are not licensed for this route of administration. Similarly, numerous combinations of drugs can be given subcutaneously. A database of compatible drug combinations is now available on the Internet (http://www.pallmed.net/).

The intravenous route is infrequently used in palliative care:[22] it is used in patients with an established central venous catheter, or when other parenteral routes are contraindicated (e.g. bleeding diathesis, poor peripheral circulation). The intramuscular route is even less frequently used in palliative care, because of the discomfort associated with intramuscular administration:[22] it is used in patients when the subcutaneous route is contraindicated (e.g. poor cutaneous circulation, irritant drug).

Management—specific problems

Airway obstruction

Airway obstruction is a common problem in patients with advanced head and neck cancer. Thus, Aird *et al.* reported an incidence of 28% amongst their cohort of patients.[23] However, airway obstruction is a relatively uncommon cause of death in head and neck cancer patients (see Table 11.1).[17]

In general, the management of airway obstruction includes treatment of the underlying cancer, performance of a tracheostomy and/or symptomatic management. However, as the disease progresses, then so the appropriateness of certain options diminishes (e.g. performance of a tracheostomy). It is important that a management plan is developed for patients at risk of airway obstruction. Moreover, it is important that the management plan is reassessed on a regular basis to take into account changes in the patient's condition. The following discussion relates to the management of airway obstruction in the terminal phase of the illness.

In cases of subacute obstruction, various interventions may be used to try to alleviate the patient's distress, e.g. corticosteroids, and helium and oxygen mixtures.[24] In addition, interventions used to treat dyspnoea itself may be of benefit in this situation, e.g. opioids, or benzodiazepines.[25]

In cases of acute obstruction, and where the patient is in extremis, a sedative drug should be used to alleviate the patient's distress, e.g. midazolam.[26] In most cases, a subcutaneous injection of 2.5–5 mg of midazolam will adequately sedate the patient. However, some patients require further/larger doses of midazolam, e.g. patients on long-term benzodiazepine therapy.

Airway obstruction is discussed in depth in Chapter 4. It should be noted that head and neck patients may have other causes of respiratory distress, including chronic obstructive pulmonary disease, lung cancer, pulmonary embolus, and aspiration pneumonia (secondary to dysphagia). Appropriate management of these problems can lead to significant relief of related symptoms (e.g. dyspnoea, cough).

Haemorrhage

Minor haemorrhages are relatively common (reported prevalence 18–47%).[17,18] However, major haemorrhages are much less common.[23] Moreover, major haemorrhages are a relatively unusual cause of death in head and neck cancer patients (see Table 11.1).[17,18]

The management of haemorrhage depends on a number of factors, including the patient's general condition/prognosis, the cause of the bleeding, the severity of the bleeding, and the sequelae of the bleeding.[27] It is important that a management plan is developed for patients at risk of haemorrhage. Moreover, it is important that the management plan is reassessed on a regular basis to take into account changes in the patient's condition. The following discussion relates to the management of haemorrhage in the terminal phase of the illness.

The management of minor/non-threatening haemorrhage may involve the use of local pressure, haemostatic dressings (e.g. alginate), topical vasoconstrictors (e.g. epinephrine), topical astringents (e.g. sucralfate), topical haemostatic agents (e.g. tranexamic acid), cauterizing agents (e.g. silver nitrate), and systemic haemostatic agents (e.g. tranexamic acid).[27,28] It is also important to correct any associated haemostatic problems, e.g. to reverse anticoagulation.

The management of major/life-threatening haemorrhage should involve the use of sedative drugs (e.g. midazolam).[29] In most cases, a subcutaneous injection of 10 mg of midazolam will adequately sedate the patient. However, some patients require further/larger doses of midazolam, e.g. patients on long-term benzodiazepine therapy. The appropriate use of midazolam does not itself alter the outcome of a bleeding episode.

Major bleeds are generally preceded by minor ('herald') bleeds. Thus, it may be possible to identify 'at risk' patients, and make preparations for such an eventuality. In such circumstances, it is recommended that the sedative drug, and other relevant items (pressure dressings, coloured blankets), are kept in close proximity to the patient.[29]

One of the major difficulties surrounding the care of patients with head and neck cancer involves the disclosure of information about the risk of airway obstruction and/or haemorrhage. It is generally appropriate to warn those patients at high risk about the possibility of such a problem occurring. Indeed, in many cases, the patient will already have considered the issue, and may be 'thinking the worst'. (In such cases, an open and honest conversation may actually help to relieve some of the psychological distress associated with these issues.) In addition, it is generally appropriate to warn the carers of those patients at high risk about the possibility of such a problem occurring. Nevertheless, in other circumstances, such conversations may in fact do more harm than good.

Support for the family

Although the focus of end-of-life care is on the patient, it is important that the needs of the family are not overlooked. Family members often require psychological/spiritual support during the terminal phase of the illness, but they may also require more practical assistance at this time (e.g. advice on legal matters/financial issues).

It is important that ongoing/future problems are identified, and that strategies are put in place to combat them. For example, it is possible to identify persons at increased risk of an abnormal bereavement reaction, and to arrange appropriate bereavement support for such persons following the patient's death.[30]

Key points

- Most head and neck cancer patients die in hospital.
- Most head and neck cancer patients die as a result of a gradual deterioration in their condition, rather than an acute event related to their condition (e.g. airway obstruction, haemorrhage).
- Most head and neck cancer patients have a relatively straightforward terminal phase.
- Patients and health care professionals may have different views about what constitutes a 'good death'.

References

1 Fardy, M. (1997). Oro-facial cancer—is there more to treatment than surgery and radiotherapy? *Palliat Care Today*, 6, 20–21.

2 Rhys Evans, P.H., and Patel, S.G. (2003). Introduction. In Rhys Evans, P.H., Montgomery, P.Q., and Gullane, P.J., eds. *Principles and practice of head and neck oncology*, pp. 3–13. London, Martin Dunitz.

3 Roodenburg, J., and Davies, A. (2005). Head and neck cancer. In: Davies, A., and Finlay, I., eds. *Oral care in advanced disease*, pp. 157–169. Oxford, Oxford University Press.

4 Doyle, D., Hanks, G., Cherny, N.I., and Calman, K. (eds) (2004). *Oxford textbook of palliative medicine*, 3rd edn. Oxford, Oxford University Press.

5 Twycross, R., Wilcock, A., Charlesworth, S., and Dickman, A. (2002). *Palliative care formulary*, 2nd edn. Abingdon, UK, Radcliffe Medical Press.

6 Walter, T. (2003). Historical and cultural variants on the good death. *Br Med J*, 327, 218–20.

7 Payne, S.A., Langley-Evans, A., and Hillier, R. (1996). Perceptions of a 'good' death: a comparative study of the views of hospice staff and patients. *Palliat Med*, 10, 307–312.

8 Steinhauser, K.E., Clipp, E.C., McNeilly, M., Christakis, N.A., McIntyre, L.M., and Tulsky, J.A. (2000). In search of a good death: observations of patients, families and providers. *Ann Intern Med*, 132, 825–832.

9 Steinhauser, K.E., Christakis, N.A., Clipp, E.C., McNeilly, M., McIntyre, L., and Tulsky, J.A. (2000). Factors considered important at the end of life by patients, family, physicians, and other care providers. *J Am Med Assoc*, 284, 2476–2482.

10 Clark, J. (2003). Freedom from unpleasant symptoms is essential for a good death. *Br Med J*, 327, 180.

11 Finlay, I.G., Higginson, I.J., Goodwin, D.M., *et al.* (2002). Palliative care in hospital, hospice, at home: results from a systematic review. *Ann Oncol*, 13 Suppl 4, 257–264.

12 Thomas, K. (2003). *Caring for the dying at home: companions on the journey*. Abingdon, UK, Radcliffe Medical Press.

13 Ellershaw, J., and Wilkinson, S. (2003). *Care of the dying: a pathway to excellence*. Oxford, Oxford University Press.

14 Shah, S.H. (2005). Integrated care pathway for the last days of life. *Palliat Med*, 19, 351–352.

15 Anonymous (1998). Cancer care during the last phase of life. *J Clin Oncol*, 16, 1986–1996.

16 Ethunandan, M., Rennie, A., Hoffman, G., Morey, P.J., and Brennan, P.A. (2005). Quality of dying in head and neck cancer patients: a retrospective analysis of potential indicators of care. *Oral Surg Oral Med Oral Pathol Oral Radiol Endod*, 100, 147–152.

17 Forbes, K. (1997). Palliative care in patients with cancer of the head and neck. *Clin Otolaryngol Allied Sci*, 22, 117–122.

18 Shedd, D.P., Carl, A., and Shedd, C. (1980). Problems of terminal head and neck cancer patients. *Head Neck Surg*, 2, 476–482.

19 Leitner, C., Rogers, S,N., Lowe, D., and Magennis, P. (2001). Death certification in patients whose primary treatment for oral and oropharyngeal carcinoma was operation: 1992–1997. *Br J Oral Maxillofac Surg*, 39, 204–9.

20 Gomes, B., and Higginson, I.J. (2006). Factors influencing death at home in terminally ill patients with cancer: systematic review. *Br Med J*, **332**, 515–518.

21 Talmi, Y.P., Bercovici, M., Waller, A., Horowitz, Z., Adunski, A., and Kronenberg, J. (1997). Home and inpatient hospice care of terminal head and neck cancer patients. *J Palliat Care*, **13**, 9–14.

22. Hanks, G., Roberts, C.J., and Davies, A.N. (2004). Principles of drug use in palliative medicine. In Doyle, D., Hanks, G., Cherny, N., and Calman, K., eds. *Oxford textbook of palliative medicine*, 3rd edn., pp. 213–225. Oxford, Oxford University Press.

23 Aird, D.W., Bihari, J., and Smith, C. (1983). Clinical problems in the continuing care of head and neck cancer patients. *Ear Nose Throat J*, **62**, 230–243.

24 Biller, J.A. (2002). Airway obstruction, bronchospasm, and cough. In Berger, A.M., Portenoy, R.K., and Weissman, D.E., eds. *Principles and practice of palliative care and supportive oncology*, 2nd edn., pp. 378–388. Philadelphia, Lippincott Williams & Wilkins.

25 Chan, K.-S., Sham, M.M., Tse, D.M., and Thorsen, A.B. (2003). Palliative medicine in malignant respiratory diseases. In Doyle, D., Hanks, G., Cherny, N., and Calman, K., eds. *Oxford textbook of palliative medicine*, 3rd edn., pp. 587–618. Oxford, Oxford University Press.

26 Regnard, C., and Hockley, J. (2004). *A guide to symptom relief in palliative care*. Abingdon, UK, Radcliffe Medical Press.

27 Friedman, K.D., and Raife, T.J. (2002). Management of hypercoagulable states and coagulopathy. In Berger, A.M., Portenoy, R.K., and Weissman, D.E., eds. *Principles and practice of palliative care and supportive oncology*, 2nd edn., pp. 452–462. Philadelphia, Lippincott Williams & Wilkins.

28 Twycross, R., and Wilcock, A. (2001). *Symptom management in advanced cancer*, 3rd edn. Adingdon, UK, Radcliffe Medical Press.

29 Lovel, T. (2000). Palliative care and head and neck cancer. *Br J Oral Maxillofac Surg*, **38**, 253–254.

30 Kissane, D.W. (2004). Bereavement. In Doyle, D., Hanks, G., Cherny, N., and Calman, K., eds. *Oxford textbook of palliative medicine*, 3rd edn., pp. 1137–1151. Oxford, Oxford University Press.

Index